SUTTER GENERAL HOSPITAL
NUCLEAR MEDICINE DEPARTMENT
2820 L STREET
SACRAMENTO, CA 95816

Multiple Imaging Procedures

IMAGING OF THE PERIPHERAL VASCULAR SYSTEM

MULTIPLE IMAGING PROCEDURES

Series Editors: Leonard M. Freeman, M.D.
Jerome H. Shapiro, M.D.

Pulmonary System
Edited by Stanley S. Siegelman, M.D., Frederick P. Stitik, M.D., and
Warren R. Summer, M.D.
Central Nervous System
Edited by Samuel M. Wolpert, M.B., B.Ch, D.M.R.D.
Abdomen
Edited by Abass Alavi, M.D., and Peter H. Arger, M.D.
Urinary Tract and Adrenal Glands
Edited by Ernest J. Ferris, M.D., and Joanna J. Seibert, M.D.
Heart
Edited by Florencio A. Hipona, M.D.
Imaging of the Peripheral Vascular System
Edited by Steven Pinsky, M.D., Gerald S. Moss, M.D.,
Siddalingappa Srikantaswamy, M.D., U. Yun Ryo, M.D., Ph.D.,
Steven A. Gould, M.D., and Gerald D. Pond, M.D.
Body Imaging in Pediatrics (*in press*)
By John R. Sty, M.D., Ramiro Hernandez, M.D., and
Richard Starshak, M.D.
Procedures in Skeletal Radiology (*in press*)
Edited by Amy Beth Goldman, M.D.

IMAGING OF THE PERIPHERAL VASCULAR SYSTEM

Editors

Steven Pinsky, M.D.

Gerald S. Moss, M.D.

Siddalingappa Srikantaswamy, M.D.

U. Yun Ryo, M.D., Ph.D.

Steven A. Gould, M.D.

Gerald D. Pond, M.D.

MULTIPLE IMAGING PROCEDURES

GRUNE & STRATTON, INC.
(Harcourt Brace Jovanovich, Publishers)
Orlando   San Diego   San Francisco   New York   London
Toronto   Montreal   Sydney   Tokyo   SãoPaulo

Library of Congress Cataloging in Publication Data
Main entry under title:

Imaging of the peripheral vascular system.

   (Multiple imaging procedures)
   Includes bibliographical references and index.
   1. Angiography.   2.   Peripheral vascular diseases—
Diagnosis.   I.   Pinsky, Steven.   II.   Series. [DNLM:
1.   Angiography.   2.   Blood vessels—Radionuclide imaging.
WG 500 I31]
RC691.6.A53I43   1984   616.1'3107575   84-4678
ISBN   0-8089-1636-X

Grune & Stratton, Inc.
Orlando, FL 32887

Distributed in the United Kingdom by
Grune & Stratton, Ltd.
24/28 Oval Road, London NW 1

Library of Congress Catalog Number 84-4678
International Standard Book Number 0-8089-1636-X
Printed in the United States of America

84 85 86 87   10 9 8 7 6 5 4 3 2 1

To our families.

CONTENTS

PREFACE

The imaging of abnormalities of the peripheral vascular system is not limited to the usual radiologic modalities. In preparing this volume, it therefore became necessary to include input from not only all of the modalities in radiology, but also from the vascular flow laboratory. Like so many other areas in diagnostic imaging, many new developments are taking place and it is difficult to remain up-to-date on all the modalities. During the course of preparation of this text, the very exciting new technique, digital subtraction angiography, was added to the modalities already being reviewed. In addition to the diagnostic modalities, we consider the radiologist's role in therapeutic angiography. In general, there are so many modalities to study the peripheral vessels that we have not attempted to recommend one modality for each pathologic condition. These modalities are so new that definitive answers on the modality of choice have not been determined. The rapid developments in all of the imaging modalities make the future of imaging of the peripheral vessels an exciting area for research. We look forward to a determination of the appropriate modality for each condition. It was our intent, however, to inform the physician about the procedures that can be used and the advantages of each of the modalities.

All too often the radiologist is not familiar with the techniques available in the blood flow laboratory, and likewise, the vascular surgeons and internists are not familiar with all the new modalities available to the radiologists. We have provided a description of all the modalities currently available to ensure that both the referring physicians and the radiologists can select the best procedure for each condition and patient.

Steven Pinsky, M.D.

CONTRIBUTORS

Carlos Bekerman, M.D.
  Clinical Staff
  Division of Nuclear Medicine
  Department of Diagnostic Radiology
  Michael Reese Hospital and Medical Center, and
  Associate Professor of Radiology and Medicine
  University of Chicago
  Chicago, Illinois

Steven A. Gould, M.D.
  Director, Blood Flow Laboratory
  Department of Surgery
  Michael Reese Hospital and Medical Center, and
  Assistant Professor of Surgery
  University of Chicago
  Chicago, Illinois

Jonathan E. Hasson, M.D.
  Surgical Resident
  Department of Surgery
  Michael Reese Hospital and Medical Center
  Chicago, Illinois

Joel Leland, D.O.
  Director, Ultrasound
  Department of Diagnostic Radiology
  Michael Reese Hospital and Medical Center, and
  Clinical Assistant Professor of Radiology
  University of Chicago
  Chicago, Illinois

Gerald S. Moss, M.D.
  Chairman, Department of Surgery
  Michael Reese Hospital and Medical Center, and
  Professor of Surgery
  University of Chicago
  Chicago, Illinois

Dushyant V. Patel, M.D.
Director, Neuroradiology
Department of Diagnostic Radiology
Michael Reese Hospital and Medical Center, and
Assistant Professor of Radiology
University of Chicago
Chicago, Illinois

Steven Pinsky, M.D.
Director, Division of Nuclear Medicine
Department of Diagnostic Radiology
Michael Reese Hospital and Medical Center, and
Associate Professor of Radiology and Medicine
University of Chicago
Chicago, Illinois

Gerald D. Pond, M.D.
Associate Professor
Department of Radiology
University of Arizona Health Sciences Center
Tucson, Arizona

U. Yun Ryo, M.D., Ph.D.
Associate Director, Division of Nuclear Medicine
Department of Diagnostic Radiology
Michael Reese Hospital and Medical Center, and
Associate Professor of Radiology and Medicine
University of Chicago
Chicago, Illinois

Janice R. L. Smith, M.D.
Assistant Professor
Department of Radiology
University of Arizona Health Sciences Center, and
Neurological Consultants
Tucson, Arizona

Siddalingappa Srikantaswamy, M.D.
Radiologist
Department of Radiology
Edgewater Hospital, and
Associate Professor of Radiology
Chicago Medical School
Chicago, Illinois

Gerald S. Moss
Steven A. Gould

1
Introduction to Vascular Imaging

Peripheral vascular surgery is a relatively new discipline. The era of modern vascular surgery began in 1948, when Gross et al.[1] published their report showing that a human arterial graft could be used to bypass a chronically diseased artery. Several years later, DuBost[2] successfully excised an abdominal aortic aneurysm and replaced it with a homograft. In 1954, Eastcott et al.[3] successfully carried out an endarterectomy of a symptomatic carotid artery stenosis. The repair of diseased peripheral arteries now constitutes one of the most common surgical procedures done in the United States and has stimulated the growth of newer and better techniques of vascular imaging.

In the early 1970s, the diagnosis of peripheral vascular disease was based on a patient history, a physical examination, and contrast arteriograms. The arteriogram has occupied a central position in the management of these patients because it generates critical anatomic information regarding inflow, run-off, the degree and extent of stenosis, and the location of adjacent vascular structures. The arteriogram, however, is often not pivotal in deciding if surgery is indicated. That decision is usually based on history and physical findings.

The history of contrast angiography began in 1896, when Haschek and Lindenthal[4] injected a viscous radiopaque solution into the blood vessels of an amputated hand. The next few decades were marked by the introduction of less viscous solutions. In the 1950s, Renografin® (Squibb) and Angio-Conray® (Malinckodt) were introduced and now enjoy universal acceptance.

The other important development in the history of contrast angiography was the development of catheter angiography. In the 1940s, angiography was carried out by direct puncture of the involved artery, such as the femoral, carotid, or the abdominal aorta, from the translumbar approach. Although satisfactory data could be obtained, the information was limited to the region of the single artery.

In 1952, Seldinger[5] introduced the catheter technique. This simple but elegant method involves the insertion of a catheter over a previously placed guide wire. Since

IMAGING OF THE PERIPHERAL VASCULAR SYSTEM Copyright © 1984 by Grune & Stratton.
ISBN 0-8089-1636-X

the catheter is the same size as the puncture hole in the artery, hemorrhage rarely occurs. This approach makes all the major vessels accessible through a single puncture in the femoral artery.

Although contrast arteriography is essential in the evaluation of patients with vascular disease, it does have disadvantages. The most important disadvantage is that it does not provide physiologic information. For example, an arteriogram may demonstrate a completely occluded superficial femoral artery, but it does not give information regarding distal perfusion pressures, which may or may not be reduced (for reasons that are not clear at present, similar patterns of arterial occlusion may be associated with quite different perfusion pressure patterns). A second drawback to arteriography is its invasive nature, which leads to several unappealing consequences: the patient must be hospitalized for these studies; the studies themselves are at least unpleasant and usually painful; arteriography generally cannot be used as a screening device for serial follow-up studies; the patient is exposed to a small but finite radiation dose; and there is a small but real risk of complications such as thrombosis or hemorrhage from the arterial puncture site. Despite these problems, arteriography remains invaluable in the management of patients with peripheral vascular disease.

Approximately 15 years ago Yao et al.[6] published papers describing the measurement of ankle systolic pressure, thereby introducing noninvasive blood flow techniques into clinical medicine. In rapid succession, techniques to measure carotid artery as well as leg vein flow dynamics were also introduced. These new noninvasive modalities have not replaced traditional arteriography, since they produce indirect anatomic information; they do, however, generate significant physiologic data. Noninvasive techniques are best used either as screening devices to identify patients who might require arteriography or in the follow-up of patients who require multiple studies over an extended period of time.

In addition, other techniques using nuclear imaging, computerized axial tomographic scanning, and digital subtraction angiography have also entered the mainstream of clinical practice. In the following chapters, we will describe how all of these modalities can be used in the diagnosis of peripheral vascular disease.

REFERENCES

1. Gross RE, Hurwitt ES, Bill AH Jr, et al: Preliminary observations on the use of human arterial grafts in the treatment of certain cardiovascular defects. N Engl J Med 239:578–579, 1948

2. Dubost C: Resection of an aneurysm of the abdominal aorta. Reestablishment of continuity of a preserved human aortic graft with result after five months. Arch Surg 64:405–408, 1952

3. Eastcott HHG, Pickering CW, Rob CG: Reconstruction of the internal carotid artery in a patient with intermittent attacks of hemiplegia. Lancet 2:994–996, 1954

4. Haschek E, Lindenthal OT: A contribution to the practical use of the photography according to Röntgen. Wein Klin Wochenschr 9:63, 1896

5. Seldinger SI: Catheter replacement of the needle in percutaneous arteriography. Acta Radiol 39:368–376, 1952

6. Yao JST, Hobbs JT, Irvine WT: Ankle systolic pressure measurement in arterial disease affecting the lower extremities. Br J Surg 56:676–679, 1969

Jonathan E. Hasson
Steven A. Gould
Gerald S. Moss

2

Blood Flow Laboratory Techniques of the Arteries

While percutaneous angiography can identify certain anatomic defects in the arterial tree, it does not provide sufficient information about the functional significance of specific lesions.[1] Doppler ultrasound, on the other hand, can be used to determine if any significant arterial occlusive disease is present; if the lesion is responsible for the symptoms; the location of the lesion; which of multiple lesions is the most significant; whether an ulcer or amputation will heal; the risk of gangrene in a limb; if a bypass or percutaneous transluminal angioplasty has been successful; and whether new symptoms are the result or a bypass or reconstruction that has failed or the result of new lesions.

Noninvasive techniques such as Doppler ultrasound and pulse volume recording thus can be used by the clinician to rapidly confirm the presence of, categorize, and evaluate the functional significance of arterial occlusive disease. Invasive arteriography can then be reserved for use in those patients in whom angioplastic or surgical intervention is deemed necessary.

DOPPLER ULTRASOUND

Technique

The Doppler effect forms the basis for the measurement of blood flow in peripheral arteries and veins. Briefly stated, the measured velocity of blood flow is proportional to the difference in frequency between sound transmitted toward and reflected from a vessel containing a moving stream of blood. Formally,

$$V_{mean} = (U \times F_d)/(2 \times F_t \times \cos \theta)$$

where V_{mean} is the mean blood flow velocity, U is the velocity of sound in the tissue

IMAGING OF THE PERIPHERAL VASCULAR SYSTEM Copyright © 1984 by Grune & Stratton.
ISBN 0-8089-1636-X

being studied, F_t is the frequency of transmitted sound, F_d is the measured difference between transmitted and received frequencies, and θ is the incident angle of sound and blood flow.

Current instruments use continuously generated and transmitted sound and are called continuous-wave Dopplers. Most instruments use a frequency of transmitted sound between 2 and 10 MHz. The frequency chosen allows the examiner to select the depth at which the blood vessel being studied can be optimally examined.

Schematically, most machines in use have transmitting and receiving crystals set at a small angle to each other in a common probe. The probe is coupled to the skin with a gel to provide better transmittance of acoustic signals. The received signal is amplified to provide an aural or graphic representation of flow velocity, which can then be recorded and measured (Fig. 2-1).

Clinically, the most useful information gathered with the use of ultrasound techniques is from the measurement of segmental limb pressures (SLPs).[2-4] Segmental limb pressures are measured by placing inflatable blood pressure cuffs at various points along the extremity to be studied and noting the pressure at which flow (the Doppler signal) returns. Since flow is presumed to start at the same time in all points of an extremity, theoretically the probe may be placed at any point distal to the cuff (ankle or wrist for convenience). The cuff should be approximately 20-percent wider than the diameter of the extremity at the point of placement in order to prevent measuring a falsely elevated pressure at which flow begins.

In a study of the lower extremity, cuffs are usually placed high and low on the thigh, at the calf, and at the ankle. Any gradient or pressure drop greater than 25 to 30 mm Hg between two adjacent levels is thought to be abnormal and to represent functionally significant disease. The brachial artery pressure is also measured. Results are expressed as absolute pressure values and in the form of ratios of the segmental

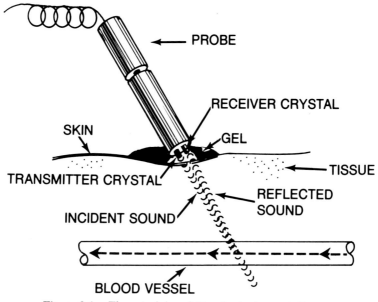

Figure 2-1. The principles of Doppler instrumentation.

Table 2-1
Normal Arterial-Brachial
Pressure Ratios

Position	Ratio
High thigh	1.0–1.2
Low thigh	1.0
Calf	1.0
Ankle	0.9–1.0

pressures (systolic) to the brachial artery pressure for normalization. Pressures may also be measured in the transmetatarsal region and at the great toe. Several investigators have also measured penile pressures in studies of vasculogenic impotence.[5] Normal ratios at the various levels along the leg are listed below in Table 2-1.

Figures 2-2, 2-3, and 2-4 give specific examples of SLP measurements found in various levels of disease.

The information gathered in the measurement of SLPs is useful in determining several of the variables mentioned in the introduction to this chapter.

The Presence of Significant Disease or Occlusion

In general, if the distal pressure ratios are greater than 0.7, vascular occlusion is not highly significant at rest and certainly is not threatening to the limb.[6] A guide to the clinical relevance of the spectrum of ankle pressure ratios is shown in Table 2-2.

Stress testing may also be performed to improve the sensitivity of segmental pressure determinations. Patients may be exercised at 2 mph at a 12-percent grade for 5 minutes or until claudication occurs. Ankle pressures are measured before and after this exercise. Presumably, the muscle bed dilates, causing increased blood flow demands in the extremity. When treadmill testing is done, lesions that are asymptomatic at rest may produce an increased and prolonged pressure drop at the ankle, indicating their functional significance with exercise.[7,8] For example, a claudicator may not demonstrate a decrease in pressure at the calf until exercised on a treadmill.

As seen in Figures 2-2, 2-3, and 2-4, the levels and functional importance of disease may be determined noninvasively with an eye toward follow-up or further investigation and surgical correction, if indicated. If ankle ratios are less than 0.2, the risk of losing a limb can be considered significant. With this information at hand, a more aggressive approach can be taken and arteriography and surgery can be employed in an attempt to salvage the limb and avoid possible amputation.[9]

Table 2-2
Ankle-Brachial Pressure Ratios

Normal	≥ 1.0
Claudication	$\leq 0.6–0.7$
Rest pain	$\leq 0.2–0.3$
Impending gangrene	≤ 0.1

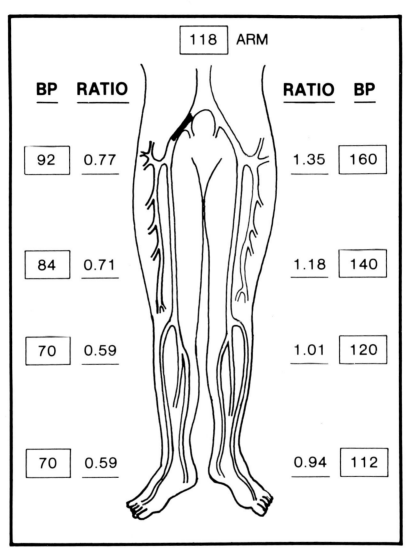

Figure 2-2. A patient with unilateral iliac occlusion exhibiting a pressure gradient at the high thigh cuff. Note the lack of gradients between other levels below the lesion.

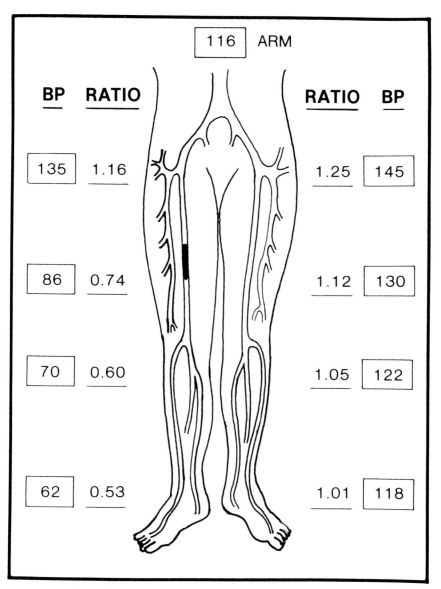

Figure 2-3. A patient with superficial femoral artery occlusion at the adductor canal exhibiting a pressure drop between the high and low thigh cuffs. There is no gradient distally.

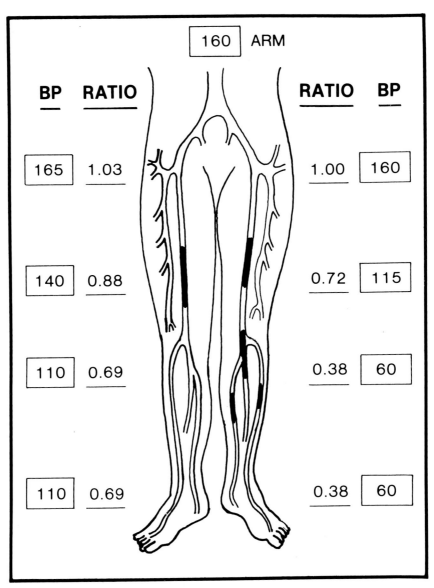

Figure 2-4. A patient with multiple levels of disease in the superficial femoral artery and in the trifurcation vessels. Note the multiple pressure gradients.

The Healing of Ulcers and Amputations

Many authors have studied the relationship between the healing of ulcers and amputations and limb pressures measured with Doppler ultrasound techniques. While there is not wide agreement on the results, a general approach can be given.

In nondiabetic patients, ulcers (ischemic) and amputation sites will generally heal (in the absence of infection) if limb pressures measured at or below the site in question are greater than 50 to 60 mm Hg. Diabetics, because of the presence of calcified, poorly compressible vessels, will often require higher pressures for healing (in the range of 70–80 mm Hg).[10] It is uncertain whether isolated toe or forefoot amputations may be safely performed at pressures below 40 mm Hg.[11,12] In all instances, however, lower pressures do not categorically exclude healing. Clinical judgment remains essential.

Correlation of Doppler studies, pulse volume recording and ^{133}Xe skin blood flow measurements has allowed more rational decisions to be made regarding the need for revascularization of extremities with nonhealing ischemic ulcers, and has permitted the rational selection of amputation sites.

Follow-up of Vascular Surgical Procedures

Intraoperative and early postoperative measurements of SLPs have been helpful in the assessment of the functional results of arterial repairs.[9,13–19] If an expected improvement in the ankle-brachial pressure ratio after bypass is not seen within 4 to 6 hours, aggressive evaluation of the patency of that bypass is indicated. In general, following femoropopliteal bypass, ankle pressures and ratios should exhibit a significant increase (a pressure ratio increase of 0.2 or more). While this may not become apparent for several hours after surgery because of various degrees of vasoconstriction and other reperfusion phenomena, the lack of significant improvement in the ankle SLP should alert the surgeon to the possibility of graft thrombosis.[16,17,20] Similarly, the sudden drop in a previously increased ankle pressure following reconstructive surgery should alert the examiner to a late onset of thrombosis.

Revascularization procedures via collateral pathways may take longer periods to produce objective improvement. While some procedures (e.g., profundaplasty, bypass to profunda arteries, femoropopliteal bypass to vessels with poor runoff) may not produce demonstrable improvement in the ankle SLP or ratio for 24 hours, failure to detect a rise at that time should stir the observer to reassess the success of the reconstruction.

It has been recommended that all patients with vascular repair or bypass be followed with frequent Doppler examinations to detect problems before graft occlusion occurs. Some of the late sequelae of bypass surgery are the development of graft stenosis, anastomotic intimal hyperplasia, and the development of new atherosclerotic lesions proximally and distally. Early recognition of these may allow correction before occlusion occurs (Figs. 2-5, 2-6).[13,14,20]

Pitfalls in the Use of Doppler Ultrasound

Several variants may cause errors in the interpretation of Doppler examinations. Significant disease in the proximal femoral artery (SFA) or profunda femoris artery may cause a low SLP in the high thigh and thus mimic iliac occlusion. Patients with calcified incompressible vessels may have falsely elevated SLPs. The presence of a large collateral vessel parallel to the one under study may give falsely elevated values. A significant stenosis with good collaterals may not produce a large gradient at rest.

The use of Doppler ultrasound techniques has been shown to be a valuable adjunct in the diagnosis and management of patients with vascular disease of the arterial system.

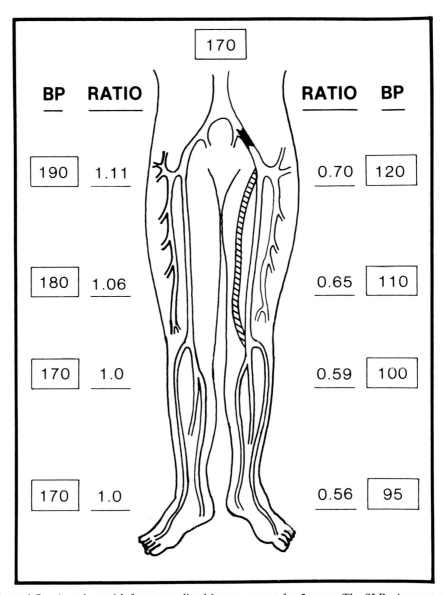

Figure 2-5. A patient with femoropopliteal bypass patent for 2 years. The SLPs demonstrate new occlusion that was confirmed by angiography to be a new iliac stenosis. The graft was still patent.

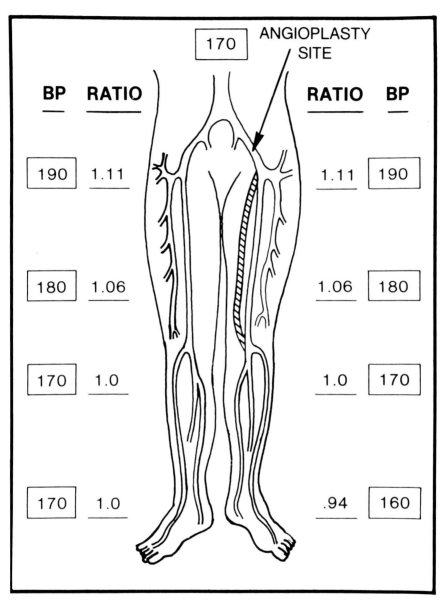

Figure 2-6. Successful balloon angioplasty of an iliac lesion.

PULSE VOLUME RECORDING

The use of the pulse volume recorder (PVR)[1] has been a major addition to the Doppler examination of the arterial system. This is a plethysmographic technique that indirectly measures the total inflow of blood into a segment of a limb. This is done by the detection of pressure and volume changes in a pneumatic cuff. A segmentally placed cuff is inflated with air to 65 mm Hg. With each cardiac cycle, the limb volume changes, and this is measured as a pressure change in the cuff. A waveform of this change is generated and analyzed. A normal tracing is shown in Figure 2-7. Standardized amplitudes of the waveforms are generated for each segment of the extremity (Table 2-3), and are shown in Figure 2-7.

The calf cuff is smaller than the thigh cuff and requires less air; the calf amplitude thus is artifactually greater than that of the thigh. This augmentation from thigh to calf is a constant finding in the presence of a patent superficial femoral artery.[18]

Pulse volume recorder tracings will vary in amplitude and contour in the presence of increasing stenosis. It can be seen in Figure 2-8 that the height of the tracing decreases and the contour becomes wider and smoother as the proximal stenosis

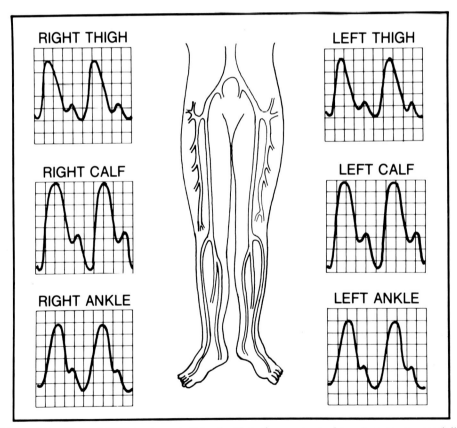

Figure 2-7. Normal PVR tracings at all levels. Note the narrow peaks and contours, especially the reflected wave or "notch" on the downstroke.

Table 2-3
Normal Pulse Volume
Recorder Amplitudes

Site	Amplitude (mm)
Thigh	≥ 15
Calf	≥ 20
Ankle	≥ 15

increases. Several specific examples of the usefulness of PVR recordings are given in Figures 2-9, 2-10, and 2-11.

Pulse volume recordings are useful as adjunctive techniques to the Doppler examination. In the case of patients with severe trifurcation disease or in those with "blind" popliteal segments, Doppler tracings may not be sensitive enough to detect significant changes in the distal tree early after reconstruction. Pulse volume recorder amplitudes and waveforms may be the only indicators of a successful bypass by demonstrating changes in pulsation of blood flow in areas inaccessible to reliable Doppler examination (Fig. 2-12)[18,19]

Pulse volume recording is a simple, rapid, painless, and useful technique, which, when used in conjunction with Doppler pressure measurements, can provide important information regarding the state of the vascular tree. The combination of PVR and

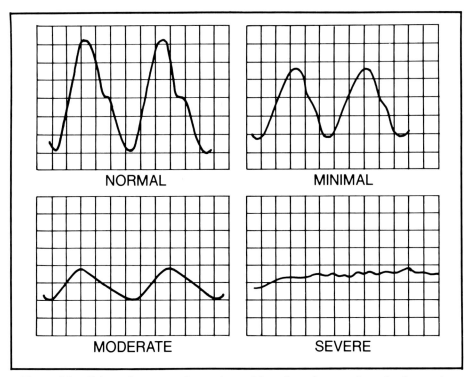

NORMAL   MINIMAL

MODERATE   SEVERE

Figure 2-8. Pulse volume recorder tracings with various degrees of proximal stenosis.

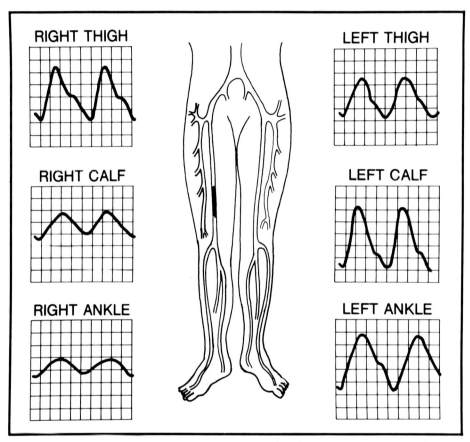

Figure 2-9. A patient with superficial femoral artery (SFA) occlusion. Note the lack of calf augmentation. This is almost diagnostic of disease in the SFA.

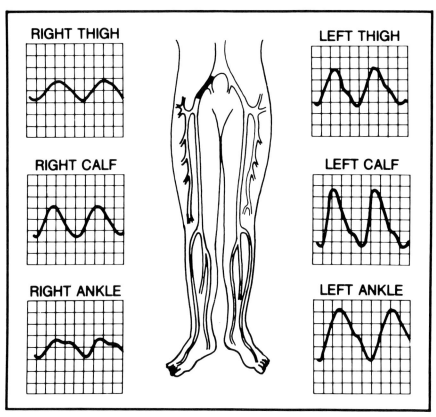

Figure 2-10. A patient with iliac stenosis. Note the decreased amplitude and widening of the tracing in the thigh. Note the augmentation of the calf PVR (patent SFA) compared with the thigh.

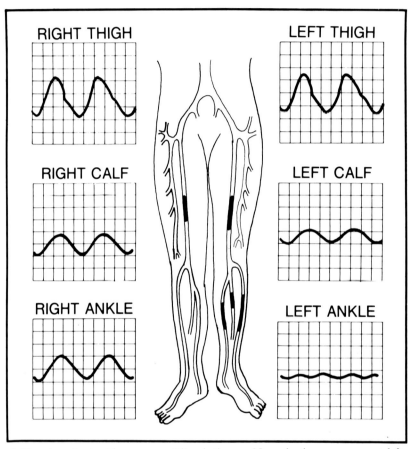

Figure 2-11. A patient with severe multilevel disease. No pulsations are seen at left ankle. The measured anklebrachial artery ratio is less than 0.1. Indication is that of severe ischemia and threatened limb loss.

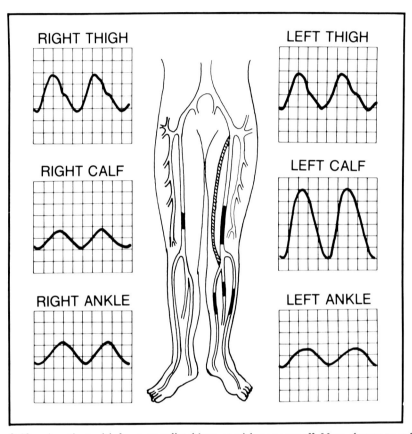

Figure 2-12. A patient with femoropopliteal bypass with poor runoff. Note change to pulsatile waveform at ankle after bypass.

Doppler techniques increases the accuracy of noninvasive diagnosis to 98 to 99 percent in the correct localization of isolated lesions when compared with arteriography.[21] These two modalities can help in the assessment, diagnosis, surgical follow-up, and prognosis of arterial disease.

REFERENCES

1. Raines JK, Darling RC, Ruth JB, et al: Vascular laboratory criteria for the management of peripheral vascular disease of the lower extremities. Surgery 79:21–29, 1976
2. Carter SA: Clinical measurement of systolic pressure in limbs with arterial occlusive disease. JAMA 207:1869–1874, 1969
3. Yao JST, Bergan JJ: Application of ultrasound to arterial and venous diagnosis. Surg Clin North Am 54:23–28, 1974
4. Yao JST: Techniques of measuring lower limb systolic pressures, in Berstein EF (ed): Noninvasive Diagnostic Techniques in Vascular Disease. St. Louis, C.V. Mosby, 1982, pp 50–56
5. Nath RL, Menzoian JO, Kaplan KH, et al: The multidisciplinary approach to vasculogenic impotence. Surgery 89:124–133, 1981
6. Yao JST: Hemodynamic studies in peripheral arterial disease. Br J Surg 57:761–766, 1970
7. Carter SA: Response of ankle systolic pressure to leg exercise in mild or questionable arterial disease. N Engl J Med 287:578–582, 1972
8. Strandness DE Jr: Exercise testing in the evaluation of patients undergoing direct arterial surgery. J Cardiovasc Surg 11:192–200, 1970
9. Goodreau JJ, Bergan JJ, Yao JST: Hemodynamic assessment of the patient with severe ischemia by Doppler ultrasound, in Bergan JJ, Yao JST (eds): Gangrene and Severe Ischemia of the Lower Extremities. New York, Grune & Stratton, 1978, pp 85–93
10. Barnes RW, Shanik GD, Slaymaker EE: An index of healing in below knee amputation: Leg blood pressure by Doppler ultrasound. Surgery 79:13–20, 1976
11. Bone SE, Pomajzl MJ: Toe blood pressure by photoplethysmography: An index of healing in forefoot amputation. Surgery 89:569–574, 1981
12. Verta MJ Jr, Gross WS, Van Bellen B, et al: Forefoot perfusion pressure and minor amputation for gangrene. Surgery 80:729–734, 1976
13. Berkowitz HD, Hobbs CL, Roberts B, et al: Value of routine vascular laboratory studies to identify vein graft stenosis. Surgery 90:971–979, 1981
14. Burnam SJ, Yao JST: Recovery room monitoring and indications for re-operation, in Bergan JJ, Yao JST (eds): Gangrene and Severe Ischemia of the Lower Extremities. New York, Grune & Stratton, 1978, pp 373–380
15. Corson JD, Johnson WC, LoGerfo FW, et al: Doppler ankle systolic blood pressure: Prognostic value in vein bypass grafts of the lower extremity. Arch Surg 113:932–935, 1978
16. Dickson AH, Strandness DE Jr, Bell JW: The detection and sequelae of operative accidents complicating reconstructive arterial surgery. Am J Surg 109:143–147, 1965
17. Garrett WW, Slaymaker EE, Heintz SE: Intraoperative prediction of symptomatic result of aortofemoral bypass from changes in ankle pressure index. Surgery 82:504–509, 1977
18. Kempczinski RF, Rutherford RB: Current status of the vascular diagnostic laboratory, in Rob C (ed): Advances in Surgery. Chicago, Year Book, 1978, pp 1–52
19. O'Donnell TF, Raines JK, Darling RC: Intraoperative monitoring using the pulse volume recorder. Surg Gynecol Obstet 145:252–254 1977
20. Yao JST, O'Mara CS, Flinn WR, et al: Postoperative evaluation of graft failure, in Bernhard V, Towne J (eds): Complications in Vascular Surgery. New York, Grune & Stratton, 1980, pp 1–19
21. Rutherford RB, Lowenstein DH, Klein MF: Combining segmental systolic pressures and plethysmography to diagnose arterial occlusive disease of the legs. Am J Surg 138:211–218, 1979

U. Yun Ryo

3
Radionuclide Studies in Arterial Disease

Radionuclide angiography has been widely used for the evaluation of vascular abnormalities. The procedure is popular because it is essentially noninvasive, uses readily available radiopharmaceuticals, and yields reliable results.[1,2]

Digital angiography, which has recently been developed will markedly reduce the need for radionuclide angiography in the future, since digital angiography is also a noninvasive procedure and the quality of the images obtained is reported to be far superior to that of radionuclide images. At present, however, digital angiography is available only at a limited number of major institutions, and the procedure is contraindicated in a considerable number of patients who are known to be allergic to contrast media. Thus, radionuclide angiography remains a convenient, simple, and effective technique for the routine evaluation of vascular diseases.

RADIOPHARMACEUTICALS

Any radionuclide with physical characteristics suitable for scintigraphy can be used for radionuclide angiography. Dynamic flow studies can be performed at the time of organ scanning, e.g., bone flow studies with ^{99m}Tc-phosphonate[3] and liver flow studies with ^{99m}Tc-sulfur colloid.[4] When static images of an anatomical abnormality are also required, a "blood pool agent," which is a radiopharmaceutical that does not leak out of the circulatory system, becomes the agent of choice.

^{99m}Tc-Human Serum Albumin

Human serum albumin (HSA) labeled with ^{99m}Tc has been used for obtaining images of the blood pool for the past two decades.[5,6] The use of this agent for the detection of aortic aneurysms was first reported by Bergan and his colleagues in 1974.[7]

IMAGING OF THE PERIPHERAL VASCULAR SYSTEM Copyright © 1984 by Grune & Stratton.
ISBN 0-8089-1636-X

Recently, ^{99m}Tc-HSA became available as a commercial kit and thus is a popular agent for cardiac function studies.[8,9]

One of the advantages of the commercial kit, which consists of lyophilized human serum albumin mixed with stannous chloride, is that it is simple to label the mixture with ^{99m}Tc-pertechnetate. With an optimum tin-HSA product and proper technique, the labeling yield can be greater than 95 percent. Another advantage of this agent is that high specific activity is easily obtainable. The high specific activity means that a good bolus injection can be made, thus the quality of dynamic flow images can be superior.

Although the quality of the blood pool images obtained with ^{99m}Tc-HSA, in general, is satisfactory, the radiopharmaceutical is less stable in the circulation than ^{99m}Tc-labeled red blood cells. One hour after an intravenous injection, an average of 62 percent of the injected dose remains in the circulation, and 34 percent remains in the circulation 4 hours after the injection.[10]

Human serum albumin is taken up and metabolized by the liver. Thus, the liver receives the highest radiation dose: 3.5 rad/10 mCi. The spleen receives 1.5 rad/10 mCi, the bone marrow receives 0.45 rad/10 mCi, and the whole-body dose is 0.16 rad/10 mCi.

[99m]Tc-Labeled Red Blood Cells

The labeling of red blood cells (RBC) with ^{99m}Tc-pertechnetate was first attempted by Fisher and his colleagues in 1967.[11] ^{99m}Tc-labeled red blood cells became a stable blood pool imaging agent when stannous chloride was introduced as a reducing agent. Two different techniques are currently available: the in vitro labeling technique and the in vivo labeling technique.

IN VITRO TECHNIQUE

Earlier techniques for in vitro labeling of red blood cells used stannous chloride, 1 μg/ml of blood mixed with the blood and incubated for 10 to 15 minutes before the ^{99m}Tc-pertechnetate was added. A specific activity of 5 mCi/ml of blood could be easily achieved.[12] A modified technique used tin-pyrophosphate, a commercial kit made for bone or myocardial infarction imaging. By using such lyophilized commercial products, the cumbersome procedures for pyrogen tests and the maintenance of sterile conditions during the preparation of the tin solution can be eliminated. It appears that the use of tin-pyrophosphate improves labeling efficiency, although the precise mechanism is not clear. The labeling procedure is relatively simple: 1 μg/ml of tin-pyrophosphate is added to 5 ml of venous blood drawn from a patient. The mixture is incubated at room temperature for 5 to 10 minutes. Then ^{99m}Tc-pertechnetate is added, and the mixture is incubated for 10 minutes. Two to three gentle agitations during the incubation period helps to improve the labeling. The yield of this modified in vitro labeling technique is greater than 90 percent. About 5 percent of the ^{99m}Tc-pertechnetate is bound to plasma protein, thus, free pertechnetate is less than 5 percent and the washing procedure can be eliminated in the labeling technique (Ryo UY: unpublished data).

IN VIVO LABELING TECHNIQUE

The in vivo labeling technique has become the most popular procedure used for cardiac blood pool imaging because it does not require the handling of blood in vitro and laboratory procedures. The procedure is simple because it involves only two venipunctures; injection of a 10 μg/kg dose of stannous ion in the form of stannous diphosphonate or pyrophosphate, followed by an injection of an optimum dose of ^{99m}Tc-pertechnetate 30 minutes later.[13]

The technique, however, has its shortcomings. Up to 15 percent of the ^{99m}Tc-pertechnetate diffuses out of the circulation immediately after the injection. The labeling yield with this technique has been reported to be over 95 percent;[14] however, the yield of 95 percent represents ^{99m}Tc-activity bound to RBCs as the percentage of activity in whole blood. The amount of ^{99m}Tc bound to RBCs as the percentage of the injected dose has not been extensively investigated in the literature.

One study compared the effectiveness of in vitro labeling and in vivo labeling in cardiac function studies.[15] The study concluded that superior images and more accurate cardiac function values were obtained with the in vitro technique.

Unlike ^{99m}Tc-HSA, ^{99m}Tc-labeled red blood cells deliver the highest radiation dose to the spleen. The radiation doses in rads from a 10 mCi dose of ^{99m}Tc-labeled red blood cells to the various organs are 1.91 to the spleen; 0.54 to the liver; 0.47 to the red bone marrow; 0.09 to the kidneys; and 0.27 to the whole body.

CLINICAL UTILIZATION OF RADIONUCLIDE ANGIOGRAPHY

Radionuclide Aortography

Radionuclide aortography is a technically simple and very reliable procedure for the detection of aortic aneurysms. Accurate detection of an aortic aneurysm with ^{99m}Tc-HSA was reported by Bergan et al.[7] in 1974. In their study, aortic aneurysms were correctly diagnosed on static blood pool images or on dynamic flow images in 26 (92 percent) of 28 patients.

Autologous red blood cells labeled with ^{99m}Tc were used for successful imaging of aortic aneurysms during the same period (Ryo et al.)[16] Recent developments in the instrumentation of ultrasonography allow accurate imaging of aortic aneurysms through simple, noninvasive techniques without radiation exposure, thus, ultrasonography currently is the procedure of choice for the detection of abdominal aortic aneurysms.[17] Digital angiography and computerized tomography are other noninvasive procedures with superior image quality that would be preferred techniques for the detection of aortic aneurysm when they are available. When a patient suspected of having an abdominal aortic aneurysm is undergoing radionuclide imaging for other purposes, a dynamic flow image of the abdomen could be obtained at the time of injection, and the abdominal aorta can be evaluated for possible aneurysmal changes.

PROCEDURE

In the majority of cases, an aortic aneurysm can be detected on dynamic flow images. The detailed location and extent of the aneurysm is, however, always better demonstrated on a static image. There is useful information that can be obtained only from dynamic flow images, such as flow interference by clot in the aneurysm and flow delay because of turbulence in the aneurysm.

A patient is positioned under a gamma camera so that the region of interest is in the field of view. When an aneurysm is suspected in the descending thoracic aorta or aortic arch, a 60-degree left anterior oblique or left lateral view flow study is more advantageous than an anterior view because the heart chambers can be separated from the thoracic aorta. A bolus injection of 10 to 20 mCi of a ^{99m}Tc-pharmaceutical is made, and the camera and dynamic imaging system or computer are activated as soon as the flow of radioactivity into the heart is visualized on a persistence scope. The recommended frame rate for the dynamic flow study is one image every 2 seconds.

After the flow study is completed, static views of the blood pool are obtained by collecting 300,000 to 400,000 counts. Multiple, anterior, oblique, and lateral views are useful for a better delineation of the extent of the aneurysm, particularly in the case of an aortic aneurysm in the chest.

DETECTION OF AORTIC ANEURYSMS IN THE CHEST

Aortic aneurysms in the chest usually produce mediastinal densities that are continuous with the aorta on a chest roentgenogram, and the diagnosis of the aneurysm can be made by radiographic findings, sometimes with the aid of fluoroscopic examination of the esophagus. These radiographic findings, however, occasionally cannot differentiate an aneurysm from other mediastinal masses.

Radionuclide angiography is a simple and effective procedure for the evaluation of a probable aortic aneurysm. Proper positioning of the patient is important for an evaluation of an aortic aneurysm in the chest. When the aneurysm is located behind the heart, an anterior view may not demonstrate abnormal flow patterns because of attenuation by the heart and superimposition of ventricular activity over the aorta.

An aneurysm will show an increased concentration of radioactivity on dynamic flow images unless it is filled with thrombus (Fig.3-1A). Static images show the aneurysm as an area of increased activity corresponding to the larger blood pool (Fig. 3-1B, white arrows). The image resolution of a radionuclide aortogram is not comparable to that of a contrast angiogram. Therefore, multiple views are necessary in order to better define the size and shape of the aneurysm. Figure 3-2 shows an example of an aortic arch aneurysm causing widening of upper mediastinum on the chest roentgenogram and deviation of the trachea. An example of an aneurysm of the ascending aorta is shown in Figure 3-3. an aneurysm of the descending aorta usually does not produce a clear abnormality on a chest roentgenogram made in the posteroanterior projection. When the probable aneurysm is best seen on a lateral view roentgenogram, the same view should be chosen for the dynamic study. When a region of increased blood pool activity is demonstrated on flow images and on static views, and the region corresponds to the suspected area on the roentgenogram, diagnosis of aortic aneurysm can be made (Fig.3-4).

Anomalous vessels sometimes cause widening of the superior mediastinum. When a soft tissuelike density is demonstrated in the superior mediastinum on a chest roentgenogram and substernal goiter is ruled out by a thyroid scintigram, a radionuclide angiogram may reveal an anomalous branch of the aortic arch to be the cause of the widened mediastinum (Fig. 3-5). Anomalous origins of the brachiocephalic trunk and subclavian artery may be seen in 10 to 20 percent of the adult population.[18]

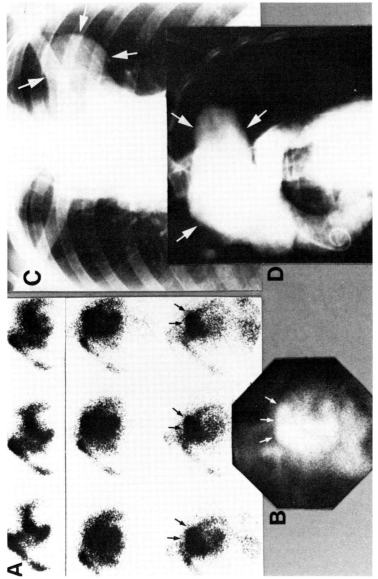

Figure 3-1. Radionuclide angiograms of a large mass in the superior mediastinum. The dynamic flow images (A) taken after a bolus injection of ^{99m}Tc-labeled red blood cells show an area of increased arterial flow in the superior mediastinum (arrows). The static image (B) shows a large aneurysmal change of the aortic arch (white arrows). The aortic aneurysm corresponds to the mass seen on the chest roentgenogram (C), and the aneurysm was confirmed by a contrast aortogram (D).

23

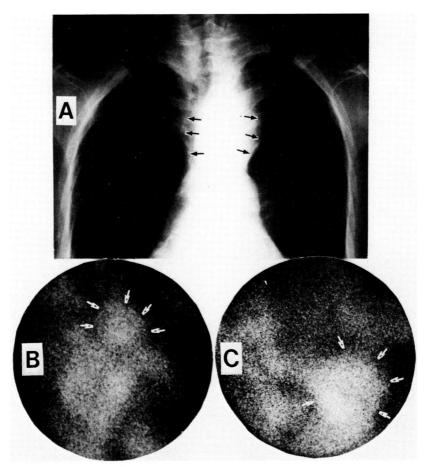

Figure 3-2. Radionuclide angiograms of a widened mediastinum. A chest roentgenogram (A) shows abnormal widening of the superior mediastinum (arrows) and deviation of the trachea toward the right. Static images (B) obtained after an intravenous injection of ^{99m}Tc-labeled red blood cells show a round aortic arch aneurysm. A magnified image (C) of the aneurysm obtained with a gamma camera equipped with a pinhole collimator shows details of the aneurysm.

DETECTION OF ABDOMINAL AORTIC ANEURYSMS

Abdominal aortic aneurysms are more easily detected than thoracic aorta aneurysms. Frequently, the disease is found by a physician incidentally during a physical examination or by the patient who discovers a pulsating mass in the abdomen.

The abdominal aortic aneurysm that is readily palpable can be confirmed by a radionuclide angiogram, and the quality of the image of the aneurysm can be often as clear as that of the contrast angiogram.

Two examples of images of abdominal aortic aneurysms on radionuclide angiograms are shown in Figure 3-6. Frequently, anterior view flow images reveal sufficient information to lead to the diagnosis of an abdominal aortic aneurysm, although the image of the aneurysm is always clearer on a static image as long as the proper

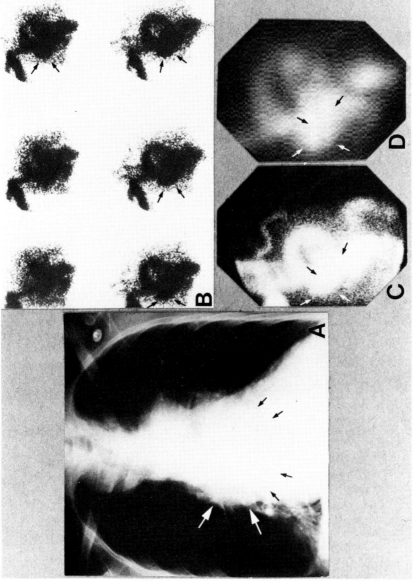

Figure 3-3. Radionuclide angiograms of an aneurysm of the ascending aorta. A chest roentgenogram (A) shows a large soft tissue density in front of the base of the heart. Dynamic flow images (B) and static analogue (C) and digital (D) images show a large aneurysm of the ascending aorta with increased blood flow and volume.

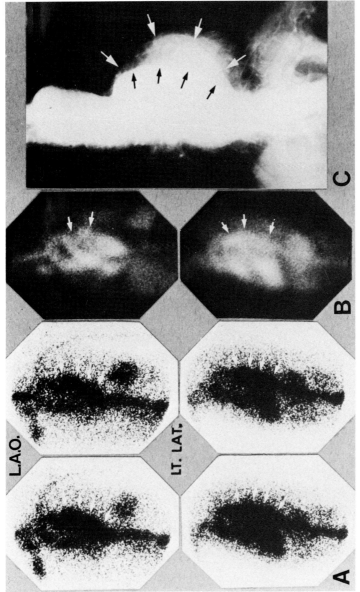

Figure 3-4. Radionuclide angiograms of an aneurysm of the descending aorta. Dynamic flow images (A) obtained in the 45-degree left anterior oblique (LAO) and left lateral (lt. lat.) views show a large fusiform aneurysm of the descending aorta (white arrows). A left lateral static image (B, bottom) shows the large aneurysm involving almost the entire descending aorta (arrows). The LAO static image (B, top), however, does not reveal the aneurysm clearly. A contrast aortogram (C) confirmed the aneurysm initially detected by the radionuclide images.

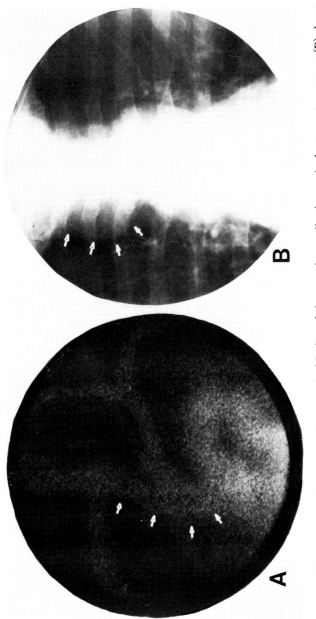

Figure 3-5. An anomalous artery that caused widening of the superior mediastinum. A chest roentgenogram (B) shows an abnormal soft tissue density in the superior mediastinum (arrows) without tracheal deviation. Substernal goiter was suggested as the probable cause of the soft tissue mass, but that possibility was ruled out after a normal thyroid scan. A static radionuclide angiogram (A) magnified by means of a pinhole collimator shows that an anomalous innominate artery was causing the soft tissue density. The innominate artery originated from the ascending aorta and branched into the right subclavian and left common carotid arteries.

27

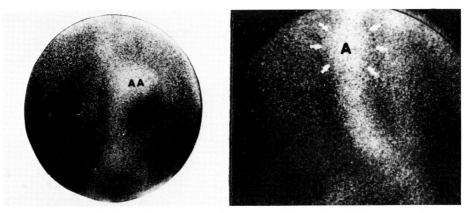

Figure 3-6. Abdominal aortic aneurysms demonstrated by radionuclide aortography. Two examples of large abdominal aortic aneurysms (AA, A) imaged with ^{99m}Tc-labeled red blood cells. The quality of the images is almost equivalent to that of contrast aortography.

radiopharmaceutical is used. When a patient with a pulsatile abdominal mass is undergoing scintigraphy of the liver, kidneys, or other organs, it is worthwhile to obtain abdominal aortic flow images at the time of injection for the evaluation of a probable aneurysm.

When aneurysmal change is extensive, a distal part of the aneurysm may not be visible on the dynamic flow images because of flow turbulence and delay proximal to the aneurysm or because of extensive thrombosis. The static images, however, always delineate the extent and configuration of the aneurysm accurately.

As mentioned earlier, ultrasonography is the procedure of choice for the evaluation of an abdominal aortic aneurysm. In certain cases, however, an ultrasonogram may detect only part of the aneurysm since the procedure usually covers the region where an aneurysm is clinically suspected. In contrast, radionuclide angiography covers areas not limited to the region of interest, thus detecting aneurysms that may not have been suspected clinically (Fig. 3-7). When the large-field-of-view camera is used, the entire abdominal aorta and iliac arteries of an average-sized adult are visible in an anterior-view abdominal angiogram.

EVALUATION OF PERIPHERAL ARTERIES

When dynamic flow studies and static imaging are properly performed, radionuclide angiography can produce very useful information on the degree of reduction of arterial flow, the presence of collateral circulation, and the efficacy of surgical intervention in the peripheral arteries. In particular, the use of computerized data-processing techniques greatly enhances the usefulness of peripheral radionuclide arteriography, since the flow rate in a particular artery can be measured semiquantitatively.

Relatively large arteries, such as the iliac, femoral, or subclavian arteries, are readily visualized on static blood pool images. Images of the venous structure can be

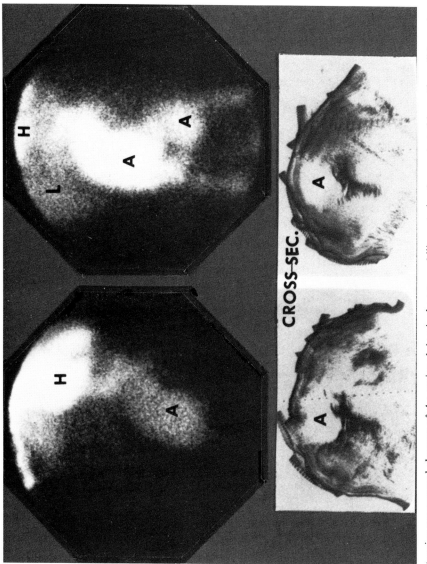

Figure 3-7. Extensive aneurysmal changes of the entire abdominal aorta and iliac arteries demonstrated by radionuclide angiography. The patient had a "pulsatile abdominal mass" for over 20 years that had recently increased in size. Ultrasonography (bottom) demonstrated a large abdominal aortic aneurysm. Radionuclide angiograms obtained with ^{99m}TC-labeled red blood cells (top) reveal extensive aneurysmal changes in the entire abdominal aorta and bilaterally in the proximal iliac arteries. An early (1 minute) blood pool image (left) shows only the aneurysm of the abdominal aorta, and a later (10 minutes) image (right) shows extensive aneurysmal changes involving the entire abdominal aorta and both iliac arteries.

29

eliminated when dynamic flow images are processed using a computer by a summing up of the flow images of the early arterial phase.

In most cases of arterial occlusive disease, flow images reveal the qualitative nature of the flow abnormality and the site of the occlusive disease (Fig. 3-8). The summation image of the arterial phase shows only the arteries, and the image reveals the area of obstruction and collateral flow. Asymmetry of the flow between the right and left arteries may be easily acknowledged on a flow image. When there is occlusive disease in the bilateral arteries, then flow through both arteries should be compared with that of an adjacent normal region such as the proximal portion of the artery above the site of the occlusion.

Semiquantitative measurement of flow rate can be done by selecting regions of interest over specific arteries and by analyzing the arterial slope of the time–activity (flow) curve (Fig. 3-9). When the curve from an abnormal artery shows a delayed peak, it is an indication of flow through collateral vessels (Fig. 3-8E).

For an evaluation of the brachial artery, radionuclide arteriography is performed only on one side at a time, since both brachial regions cannot be included in the field of view of even a large-field-of-view camera. In such cases, flow through the diseased artery should be compared with the flow of an adjacent normal artery, e.g., the ipsilateral carotid artery (Fig. 3-10). When radionuclide arteriography is performed on an arm, it is important to remember that injection of radionuclide should be made into a vein of the contralateral arm, since in the majority of cases, some degree of stasis of the radioactivity occurs in the injected vein.

The spatial resolution of scintigraphic images is not high enough to detect abnormalities in smaller arteries, in general, but an artery as small as a radial or ulnar artery can be clearly identified on a summation flow image of the arterial phase (Fig. 3-11). Visualization of these arteries allows an accurate selection of regions of interest, thus making demonstration of the flow rate in each artery possible. In the lower extremity, accurate evaluation of arterial flow can be done in anterior and posterior tibial arteries (Fig. 3-12).

Aneurysms of the smaller arteries are also readily detected by radionuclide arteriography. The aneurysm is delineated on a static blood pool image even when there is a partial obstruction of flow because of thrombosis or intimal atheroma distal to the aneurysm (Fig. 3-13).

Radionuclide angiographic technique has also been effectively utilized for the evaluation of the peripheral circulation and tissue perfusion. Using ^{99m}Tc-labeled red blood cells, Raynaud's phenomenon can be evaluated by measuring the radioactivity in the hand and the fingers, which represents blood volume, and monitoring the changes before, during, and after cold exposure.[19] By using the labeled RBCs, the blood volume of the hand and its changes can be monitored for several hours, thus, evaluation of the peripheral circulation before and after an intervention becomes possible without additional injections of radionuclide.

On the other hand, successful evaluation of peripheral vascular injuries has been done by using ^{99m}Tc-pertechnetate, ^{99m}Tc-sulfur colloid, or ^{99m}Tc-labeled red blood cells in the assessment of traumatic arterial injury or of reconstructive hand surgery.[20,21] In the assessment of arterial injury, radionuclide angiography was found to be as specific as contrast angiography[20] and probably more sensitive in demonstrating the status of tissue perfusion.[21]

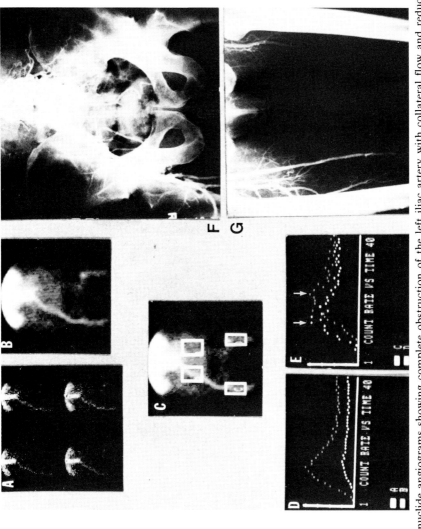

Figure 3-8. Radionuclide angiograms showing complete obstruction of the left iliac artery with collateral flow and reduced flow through the right iliac artery. The flow images (A) show an absence of early arterial flow in the left iliac artery. The flow in the right iliac artery appears to be markedly decreased compared with flow in the abdominal aorta. A static image (B) reveals markedly decreased left iliac arterial flow and collateral flow reaching the proximal femoral artery. The findings are confirmed by the time-activity curves generated from the right and left iliac (D) and femoral artery (E) regions. Contrast angiograms (F,G) later confirmed the extensive arterial disease detected initially by the radionuclide angiograms.

31

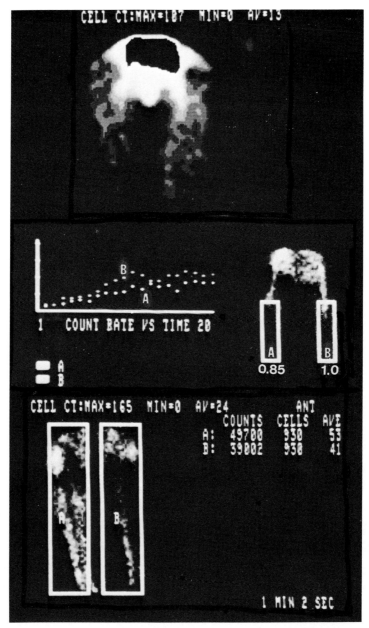

Figure 3-9. A semiquantitative evaluation of an arterial flow abnormality with radionuclide angiography. Arterial flow in the right thigh was compared with flow in the left thigh by means of the slopes of the time–activity curves (middle) generated by a computer from the regions over the right (A) and left (B) femoral arteries.

By measuring the arterial slopes, the relative flow rate can be compared between the right and left tibial arteries. The radioactivity count accumulated during the arterial phase over the region of interest (bottom) represents relative blood volume in the region during the given time.

32

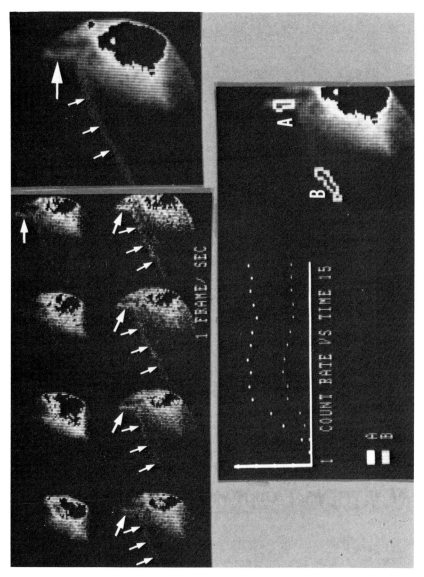

Figure 3-10. Radionuclide angiograms of the right shoulder and arm showing the axillary and brachial arteries. The flow in the brachial artery appears to be decreased on the flow images (small arrows). The decreased flow could be confirmed by comparing (bottom) the brachial flow to that in an adjacent normal artery, in this case the right carotid (large row).

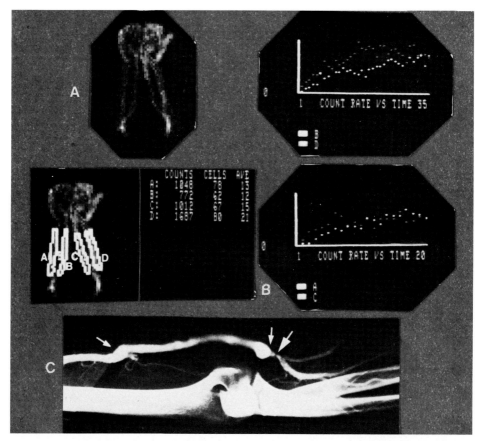

Figure 3-11. Radionuclide angiograms of the radial and ulnar arteries. From the dynamic flow images stored in a computer, images of the arteries without superimposed veins were constructed by summing up the early arterial phase flow images (A). From this reconstructed arterial image accurate regions of interest were drawn for the measurement of relative flow rates in the smaller arteries (B, left). The patient shown here had developed thrombosis of the radial artery after a cardiac catheterization and underwent brachial-radial artery grafting with subsequent development of stricture at the distal end of the anastomosis (C, contrast arteriogram).

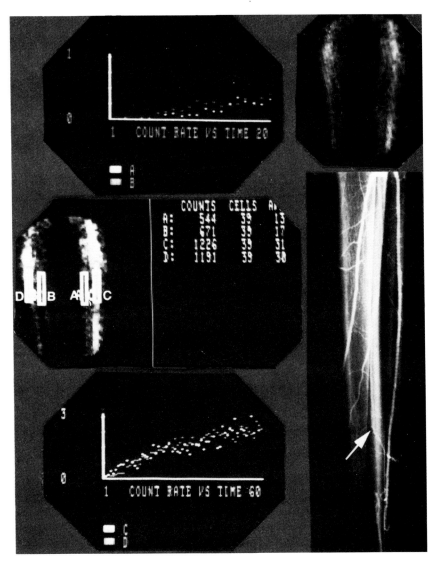

Figure 3-12. Radionuclide angiograms of the tibial arteries. The posterior and anterior tibial arteries are readily identifiable on the "summed arterial phase" image (top right). The arterial flow slope (top left) obtained from the regions over the tibial arteries (middle left) showed decreased flow in the region of the left anterior tibial artery. The contrast angiogram (bottom right) showed obstruction of the anterior tibal artery (arrow).

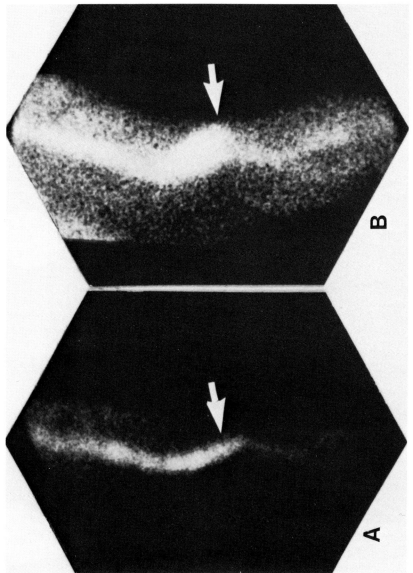

Figure 3-13. Peripheral radionuclide angiograms demonstrating a popliteal artery aneurysm. The early arterial image (A) shows a partial obstruction of the distal popliteal artery with sudden narrowing of the flow (arrow). The delayed image (B), however, shows an aneurysm of the popliteal artery that corresponds to a palpable, pulsatile, soft mass in the popliteal fossa. Arterial flow in the tibial artery is markedly decreased because of stenosis of the artery distal to the aneurysm.

REFERENCES

1. Ryo UY, Pinsky SM: Radionuclide angiography with 99m-technetium-RBCs. CRC Crit Rev Clin Radiol Nucl Med 8:107–128, 1976
2. Muroff LR, Freedman GS: Radionuclide angiography. Semin Nucl Med 6:217–230, 1976
3. Maurer AH, Chen DCP, Camargo EE, et al: Utility of three-phase skeletal scintigraphy in suspected osteomyelitis. J Nucl Med 22:941–949, 1981
4. Sarper R, Fajman WA, Tarcan YA, et al: Enhanced detection of metastatic liver disease by computerized flow scintigram. J Nucl Med 22:318–321, 1981
5. McAfee JG, Stern HS, Fueger GF, et al: 99mTc-labeled serum albumin for scintillation scanning of the placenta. J Nucl Med 5:936–946, 1964
6. Webber MM, Tobin PL, Bennett LR: Cardiac blood pool scanning with technetium-99m pertechnetate labeled albumin. Radiology 87:867–871, 1966
7. Bergan JJ, Yao RST, Henkins RE, et al: Radionuclide aortography in the detection of arterial aneurysms. Arch Surg 109:80–83, 1974
8. Chervu LR: Radiopharmaceuticals in cardiovascular nuclear medicine. Semin Nucl Med 9:241–256, 1979
9. Treves S: Detection and quantitation of cardiovascular shunts with commonly available radionuclides. Semin Nucl Med 10:16–26, 1980
10. Henkin RE: Radiopharmaceuticals for radionuclide angiography, in Siegel M, Ryo UY (eds): Evaluation of Vascular Disease: Nuclear Medicine. Cleveland, CRC Press, 1984, (in press)
11. Fisher J, Wolf R, Leon A: Technetium-99m as a label for erythrocytes. J Nucl Med 8:229–232, 1967
12. Ryo UY, Mohammadzadeh AA, Siddiqui A, et al: Evaluation of labeling procedures and in vivo stability of 99mTc-red blood cells. J Nucl Med 17:133–136, 1976
13. Stokely EM, Parkey RW, Bonte FJ, et al: Gated blood pool imaging following 99mTc stannous pyrophosphate imaging. Radiology 120:433–434, 1976
14. Pavel DG, Zimmer AM: In vivo labeling of red cells with 99mTc: A new approach to blood pool visualization. J Nucl Med 18:305–308, 1977
15. Hegge FN, Hamilton GW, Larson SM, et al: Cardiac chamber imaging: A comparison of red blood cells labeled with Tc-99m in vitro and in vivo. J Nucl Med 19:129–134, 1978
16. Ryo UY, Lee JI, Zarnow H, et al: Radionuclide angiography with 99mTc-labeled red blood cells for the detection of aortic aneurysm. J Nucl Med 15:1014–1017, 1974
17. Goldberg BB: Abdominal aorta, in Gottlieb S, Viamonte Jr. (Eds): Diagnostic Ultrasound. American College of Radiology, 1972, pp 60–62
18. Warkany J: Congenital malformations. Chicago, Year Book, 1971, p 529
19. Ryo UY, Siddiqui A, Ellman MH, et al: A study on usefulness of Tc-99m-RBC for an evaluation of hand blood flow in patients with Raynaud's phenomenon, abstracted. J Nucl Med 17:564, 1976
20. Rudavsky AZ, Moss CM: Radionuclide angiography for the evaluation of peripheral vascular injuries, in Freeman LM, Weissman HS (eds): Nuclear Medicine Annual. New York, Raven Press, 1981, pp 315–335
21. Agress H Jr, Rauscher GE, Bikoff DJ: The value of radionuclide angiography in the management and prognosis of microsurgically reconstructed digits. J Nucl Med 23:26, 1982

Siddalingappa Srikantaswamy
Joel Leland

4

Plain Film, Ultrasound, and Computed Tomographic Studies of Arteries

PLAIN FILMS

Routine plain x-ray films may not by themselves be an aid in diagnosing vascular disease, but an occasional vivid roentgenographic presentation can alert the radiologist to suspect serious vascular lesions.

The patchy calcifications of atheromas (Fig. 4-1) or the smooth uninterrupted calcifications seen in medial calcific sclerosis, hyperparathyroidism, and diabetes (Figs. 4-2, 4-3) are very familiar radiologic observations. Although the lumen is patent, in medial calcific sclerosis, the calcified vessel is highly vulnerable to trauma (Fig. 4-2). Likewise, the radiologically apparent calcified walls of an aneurysm may alert the radiologist to the presence of a clinically unsuspected aneurysm (Figs. 4-4, 4-5).

The diagnosis of aortic dissection is strongly aided by the appearance of an increased distance between the intimal calcification and the aortic border (Fig. 4-6), which is an occasional finding during the interpretation of chest films.

Calcified thrombi in the veins alert the radiologist to the possibility of chronic venous insufficiency (Fig. 4-7). Likewise, phleboliths at unfamiliar locations aid the radiologist in diagnosing unusual vascular lesions (Fig. 4-8). Heterotopic metaplastic subcutaneous ossifications are the end result of the chronic venous insufficiency seen in elderly patients (Fig. 4-9).

The observation of an obliterated margin of the psoas muscle in the proper clinical setting instantaneously leads to a diagnosis of a leaking abdominal aortic aneurysm (Fig. 4-10).

Another fascinating and classical sign of an aortic aneurysm is the erosion of the anterior borders of the vertebral bodies. Dramatic presentation of a mycotic aneurysm with perivascular gas collection on a plain film is clinically invaluable and unforgettable.

IMAGING OF THE PERIPHERAL VASCULAR SYSTEM Copyright © 1984 by Grune & Stratton.
ISBN 0-8089-1636-X

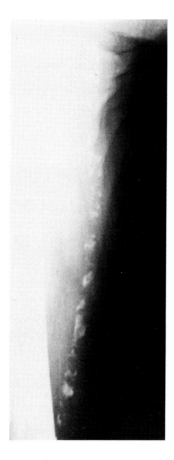

Figure 4-1. Patchy calcifications of an atherosclerotic superficial femoral artery.

ULTRASOUND

Gray scale ultrasound is a useful and accurate screening procedure for identifying and assessing the morphologic features of the abdominal aorta[1-3] and the peripheral arterial vessels of the lower extremities.[4-7] It is rapid, noninvasive, and demonstrates the true size of the vessel and not just the blood filled lumen of aneurysms. A diagnostic accuracy of 98 percent in the evaluation of pulsatile abdominal masses has been reported.[8,9]

B-mode ultrasonography is a definitive diagnostic tool in assessing abdominal aortic aneurysms.[3] Scans of the aorta are obtained in the longitudinal and transverse planes. This allows assessment of the maximum diameter of the vessel. Longitudinal scans should be oriented in the plane of the aorta. This becomes more difficult in a patient with an ectatic aorta. The aorta can be demonstrated from the left ventricle to the bifurcation, but on occasion bowel gas will present a problem by obscuring portions of the aorta, particularly the distal portion (Fig. 4-11).[1] A technique for visualizing the bifurcation by placing the patient in the left lateral decubitus position and scanning through the liver has been described (Fig. 4-12).[10] This can be helpful in the presence of bowel gas.

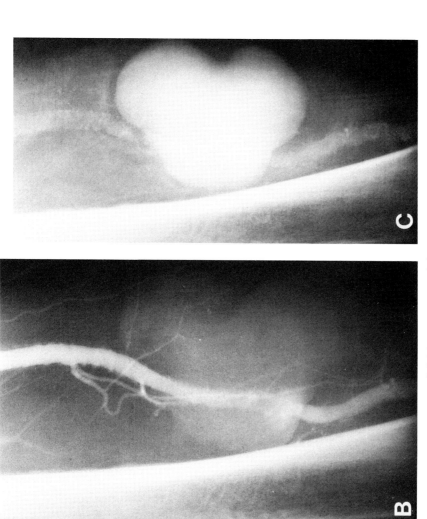

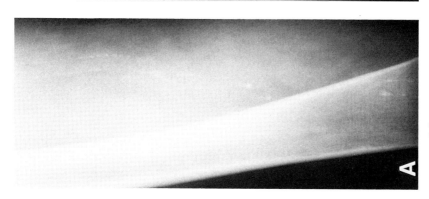

Figure 4-2. (A) Smooth continuous medial calcification of the superficial femoral artery. (B) A patent lumen with periarterial extravasation because of traumatic fracture of the vessel wall. (C) Complete opacification of a pseudoaneurysm.

41

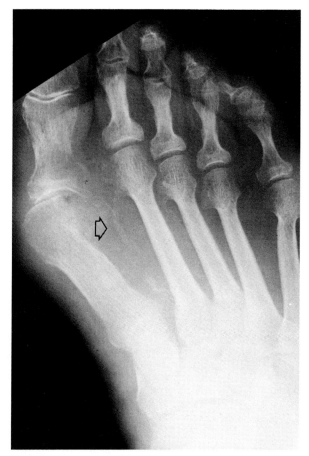

Figure 4-3. Calcifications of the branches of the dorsalis pedis artery branches in a diabetic individual.

The development of high resolution real-time units has been particularly helpful in evaluating the abdominal aorta. The plane of the aorta can easily be found and the true character of a tortuous aorta can be outlined. The pulsatile nature of the vessel can be studied and para-aortic masses can be easily differentiated (Fig. 4-13). A dissecting abdominal aortic aneurysm can be diagnosed on real-time scans by visualizing the undulating intimal flap, which can be missed on a static B-scan (Fig. 4-14).[9] Gentle pressure with the real-time probe may be helpful in displacing bowel gas.

Static B-scanning lends itself well to evaluation of the femoral, popliteal, and iliac vessels. The femoral arteries are best demonstrated in the transverse plane in the inguinal region with the patient supine. The popliteal vessels are studied in longitudinal and cross-section with the patient prone. Palpation of the vessel is helpful in determining its course.

The ability of ultrasound to aid in the diagnosis of abdominal aortic aneurysms has been well established.[2,3] Ultrasound can define the size of an aneurysm in its

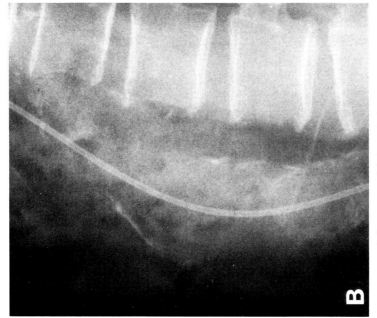

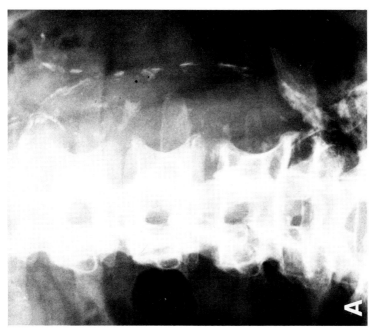

Figure 4-4. Calcifications of the walls of aortic aneurysms. (A) AP view (B) lateral view.

43

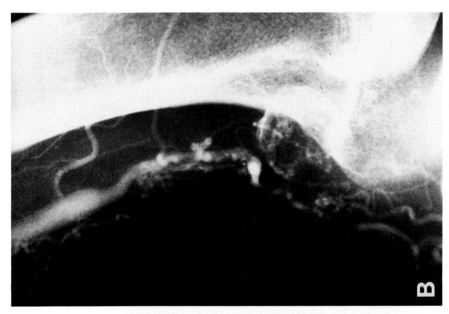

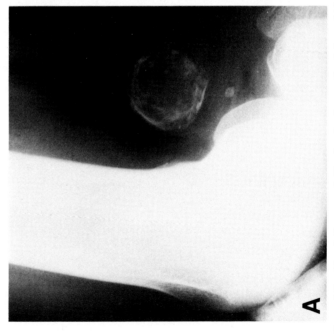

Figure 4-5. Eggshell type calcification in the popliteal fossa (A). The arteriogram (B) reveals occlusion of the popliteal artery as a result of a thrombosed aneurysm.

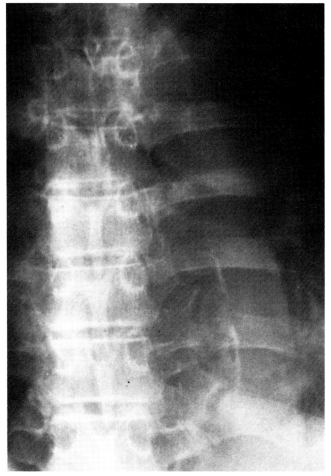

Figure 4-6. Unusual medial location of an intimal calcification in relation to the aortic wall in a patient with aortic dissection.

entirety; not only the lumen, but also the actual size of the entire vessel can be precisely measured (Fig. 4-15). Ultrasound frequently will demonstrate an aneurysm to be larger than that demonstrated on an aortogram because of intraluminal clot, which cannot be detected by aortography (Fig. 4-16). Three centimeters is considered the lower limit for aneurysmal dilatation of the aorta.

In addition to aneurysms, ultrasound can detect a normal aorta with an overlying mass (see Fig. 4-12). The transmitted pulsation can simulate an aneurysm on physical examination. A tortuous aorta can be defined, particularly with real-time scanning. In thin patients, the aorta can lie anteriorly and can produce a pulsatile mass (see Fig. 4-11).

The relationship of abdominal aortic aneurysms to the renal arteries is of critical importance and affects the type of surgery as well as the morbidity and mortality of the operation. Although 95 percent of abdominal aortic aneurysms begin below the level of the renal arteries, aortography is almost always performed to demonstrate this relationship. Demonstration of the renal arteries in relationship to the aneurysm

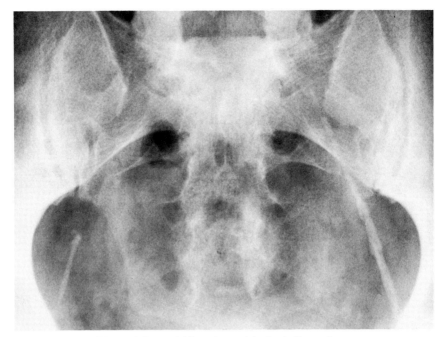

Figure 4-7. Calcified thrombi in both iliac veins.

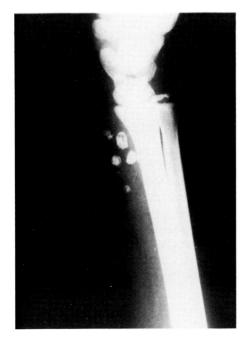

Figure 4-8. Phleboliths in soft tissues caused by an hemangioma.

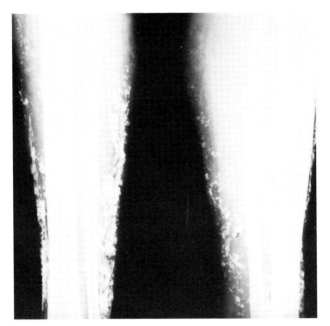

Figure 4-9. Subcutaneous metaplastic ossification in a patient with chronic venous insufficiency.

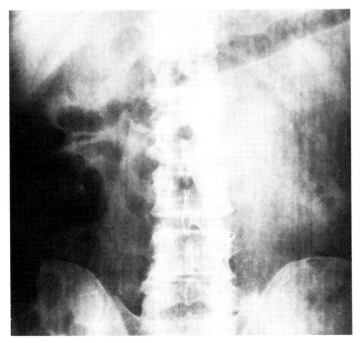

Figure 4-10. Obliteration of the left psoas margin caused by a leaking abdominal aortic aneurysm.

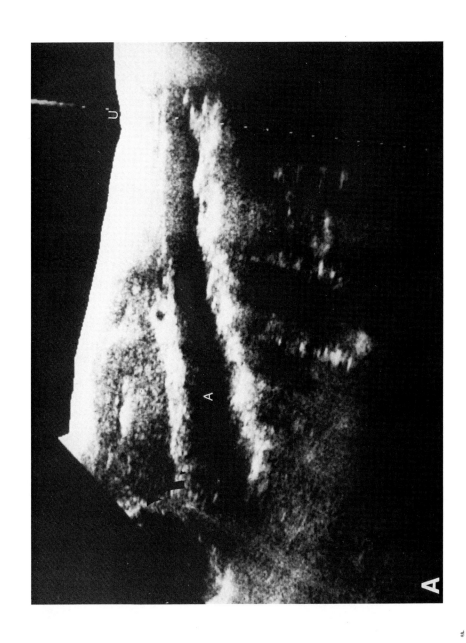

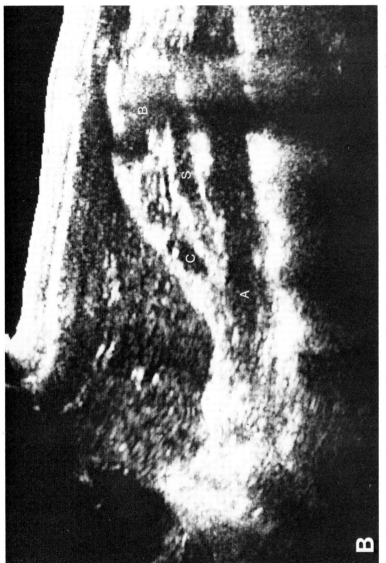

Figure 4-11. Longitudinal scan of the aorta (A) from the diaphragm (arrow) to the umbilicus (U). Note the anterior location of the distal aorta. (B) Longitudinal scan of the aorta. A portion of the aorta is obscured by bowel gas. A = aorta; C = celiac axis; S = superior mesenteric artery; B = bowel.

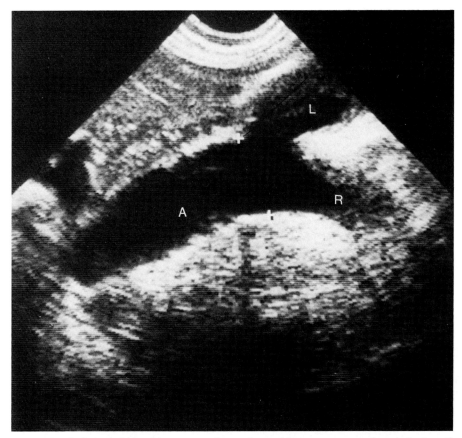

Figure 4-12. Left lateral decubitus scan of a patient with an aneurysm demonstrating the bifurcation. A = aorta; L = left iliac artery; R = right iliac artery.

by ultrasound would obviate the need for aortography. A technique utilizing a 45-degree or 70-degree LPO position has been described for demonstrating the renal arteries on B-scans.[11] The renal arteries can also be detected using real-time scanning and scanning transversely through the renal hilum and tracing the vessel to the aorta. The renal arteries lie posterior to the renal veins (Fig. 4-17). The superior mesenteric artery is more easily demonstrated than the renal arteries, and its location on a longitudinal scan can be useful, since the renal arteries arise only 1 to 2 cm below the superior mesenteric artery. If the superior mesenteric artery can be demonstrated to be at least 4 cm above the aneurysm, then a diagnosis of an aneurysm arising from below the renal arteries can be made with confidence (Fig. 4-18). Extension of an abdominal aortic aneurysm into the iliac arteries can also be demonstrated with ultrasound by longitudinal and transverse scans at and below the bifurcation (Fig. 4-19).

Prosthetic vascular grafts can be evaluated with ultrasound and the patency of the graft defined.[12] The junction of the graft and the aorta can usually be demonstrated. Complications of vascular grafts including pseudoaneurysms, fluid collections around the graft, hematomas (Fig. 4-20), and abscesses (Fig. 4-21) can also be detected.[13] These are seen as echo-free masses around the graft.

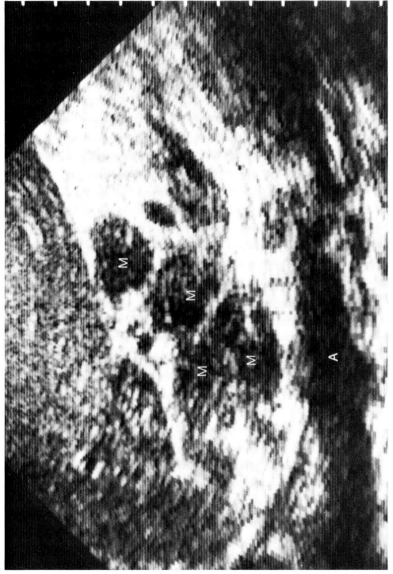

Figure 4-13. Longitudinal scan of a patient with non-Hodgkin's lymphoma who had a pulsatile pulsitic mass, which proved to be a preaortic lymph node. A = aorta; M = lymph node.

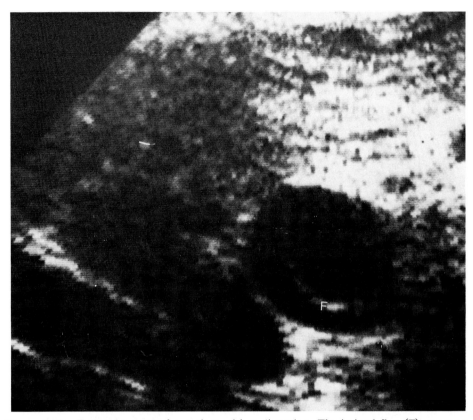

Figure 4-14. Transverse scan of a patient with a dissection. The intimal flap (F) was seen undulating on real-time scanning.

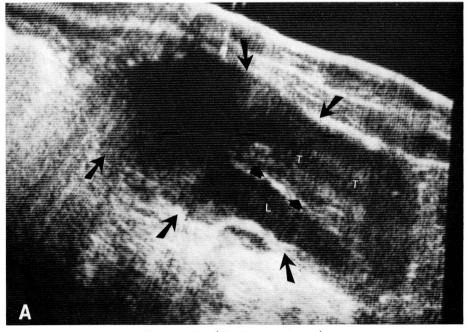

Figure 4-15. (*Continues next page.*)

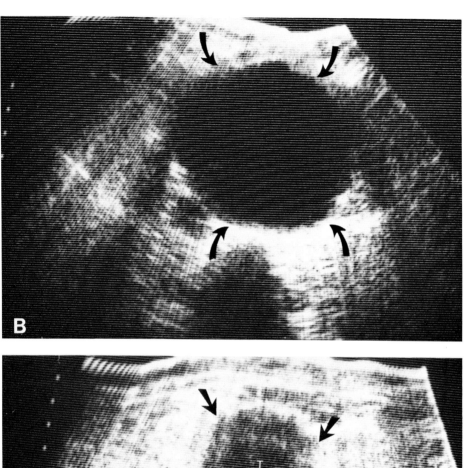

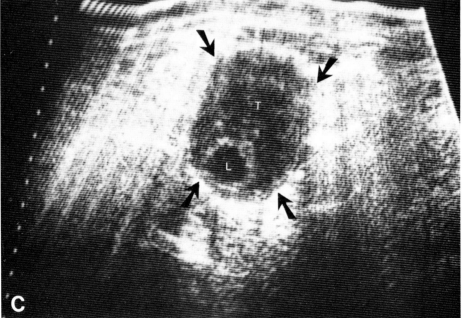

Figure 4-15. (A) Longitudinal scan of an abdominal aortic aneurysm (arrows) with thrombus (T) in the distal portion (arrow heads). L = distal aortic lumen. (B) Transverse scan through the proximal portion of the aneurysm (arrows). (C) Transverse scan through the distal portion of the aneurysm (arrows). T = thrombus; L = lumen of aorta.

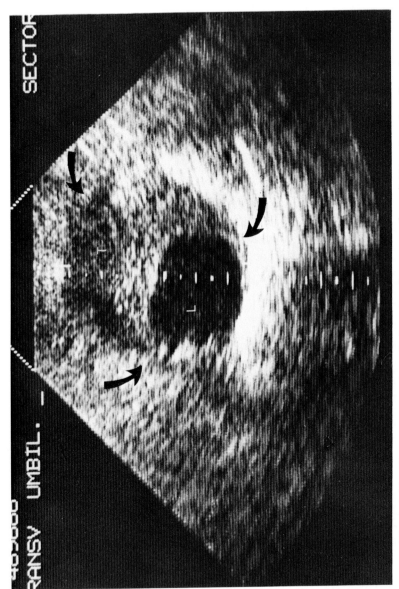

Figure 4-16. Transverse scan through thrombosed aneurysm (arrow). T = thrombus; L = lumen.

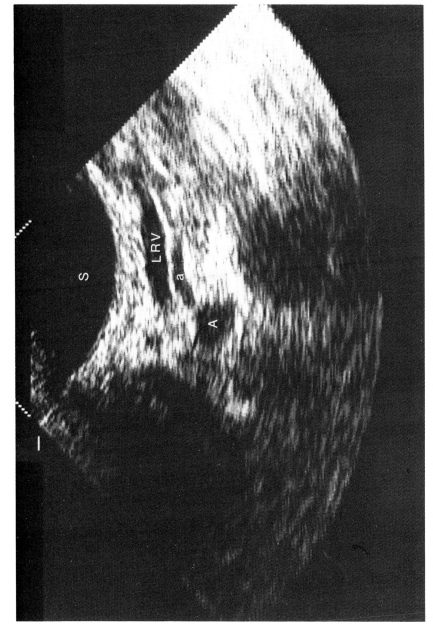

Figure 4-17. Real-time scan done transversely through the left renal hilum showing the aorta (A), the left renal vein (LRV), and the left renal artery (a) Note the fluid-filled stomach (S).

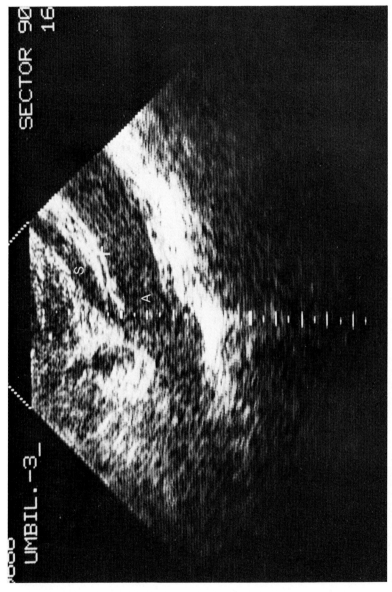

Figure 4-18. Longitudinal scan through proximal artery (in the same patient as shown in Fig. 4-16) showing the normal caliber of the proximal aorta (A) and the superior mesenteric artery (S).

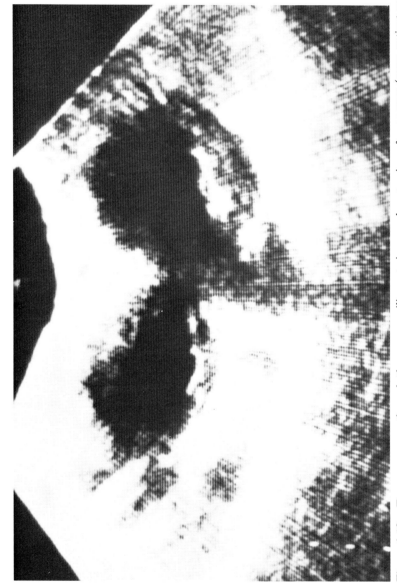

Figure 4-19. Transverse scan through the common iliac arteries reveals extension of aneurysm (same patient as shown in Fig. 4-15).

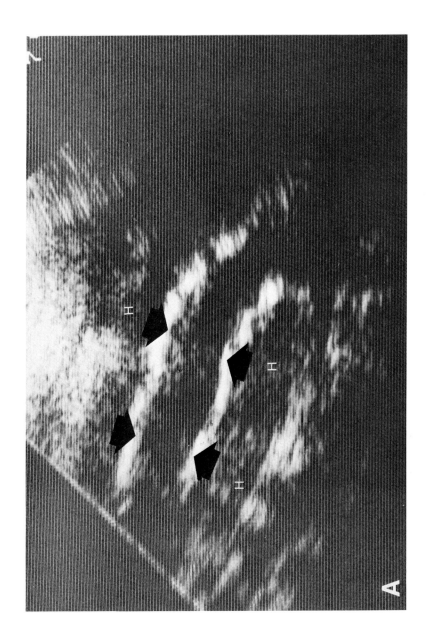

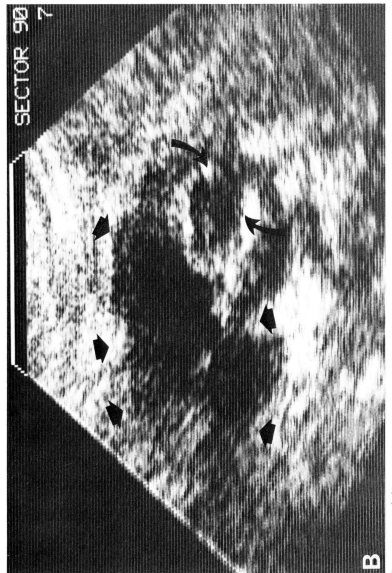

Figure 4-20. (A) Longitudinal scan of femoral portion of a femoral-popliteal bypass graft (arrowheads) with a mass representing hematoma (H) surrounding the graft. (B) Transverse scan of the graft (arrows) and hematoma (arrowheads).

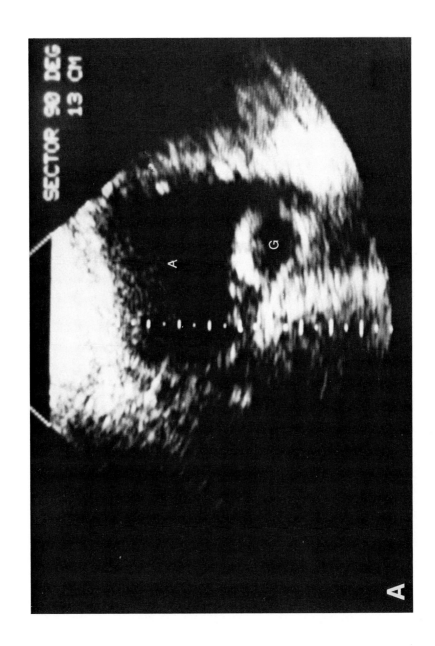

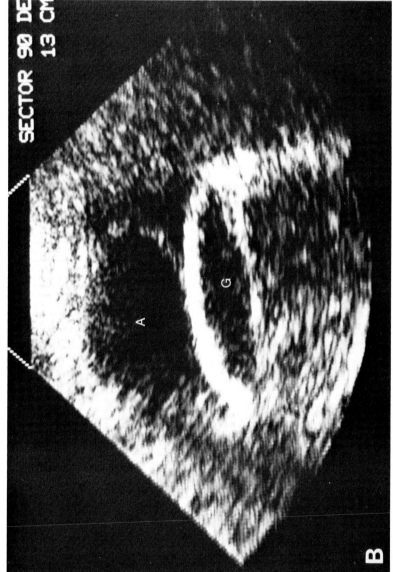

Figure 4-21. Transverse (A) and longitudinal (B) scans of a patient with a vascular graft of the femoral artery complicated by abscess. G = graft, A = abscess.

False aneurysms are pulsating hematomas connected to an arterial lumen. The inguinal area is the most common site for graft complications, but they may appear anywhere secondary to trauma (Fig. 4-22A,B,C). The popliteal artery is the most common site for peripheral artery aneurysms, accounting for 70 percent of peripheral aneurysms.[14] They occur in the sixth and seventh decade, and are bilateral in 50 percent of cases;[5] atherosclerosis is usually the cause. A sonolucent mass, occasionally with evidence of thrombus, will be seen. Continuity with the proximal or distal artery is helpful in the diagnosis and also to rule out a popliteal cyst.

Ultrasound can detect thrombus within the aneurysm and give an accurate estimate of size. An advantage of ultrasound over arteriography is its ability to detect an aneurysm in the presence of a proximal occlusion.[6]

COMPUTERIZED AXIAL TOMOGRAPHY

Computerized axial tomography (CT) is an accurate and noninvasive modality for obtaining direct images of the major vascular structures. The radiographic exploration of the retroperitoneal anatomy[15,16] has been further reinforced with the assistance of CT. In many individuals generous amounts of retroperitoneal fat aids in the sharp definition of the vessels, perivascular spaces, and the retroperitoneal compartments.

Use of CT is helpful in evaluating the presence and the physical dimensions of an aneurysm of the aorta.[17,18] The presence of mural thrombi calcifications are shown to better advantage (Figs. 4-23, 4-24). Mural thrombi are a limitation to contrast angiography. Like ultrasound, CT scanning detects the presence and extent of the aneurysm.[19–22] It also detects the presence of hemorrhage from a leaking aneurysm. Unlike ultrasound, CT has the advantage of better delineation of the aneurysm from the neighboring structures. It can also be used as a guide in tracing the pathways of the extravasated blood (Fig. 4-25). Such pathways include bleeding into the retroperitoneum, the inferior vena cava, the psoas muscle, the duodenum, or even into the peritoneal cavity.[23–28] It should be recognized that the attenuation values of the hematoma are time dependent.[29] As the hematoma ages, there is a lowering of the initial higher attenuation values. Such lower attenuation values can also be possessed by other incidental processes, such as adenopathy, fibroses, abscesses, and other necrotic neoplasms. In such instances, CT by itself cannot differentiate the histologic contents of the periaortic process, especially in the presence of an aneurysm (Fig. 4-26).

Although CT can be used as a guide in making a diagnosis of dissections of the aorta,[30] contrast aortography is mandatory before surgery. With the help of CT, evaluation of mycotic vascular lesions[31] (Fig. 4-27), thrombosed aneurysms (Fig. 4-28), pseudoaneurysms (Fig. 4-29), and calcified intravascular thrombi (Fig. 4-30) can be better demonstrated. Computed tomography is extremely helpful in evaluating postoperative patients, especially to demonstrate the presence of infections, leaks, and abnormal communications.

Standard Technique

Before CT evaluation, a history of allergic reactions to intravenous infusion of radiographic contrast media should be elicited. In supine projections, body sections of the abdomen are obtained at 2-cm intervals from the xiphoid process to the level

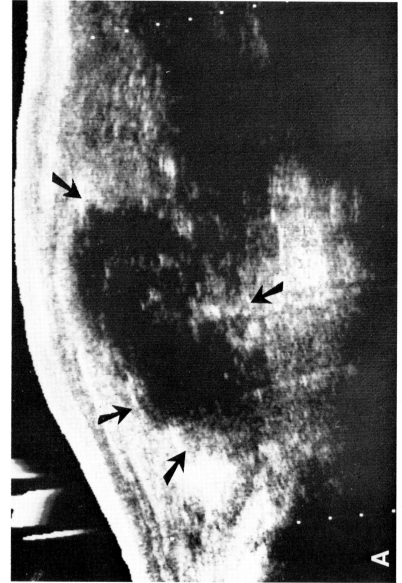

Figure 4-22. (*Continues next page.*)

63

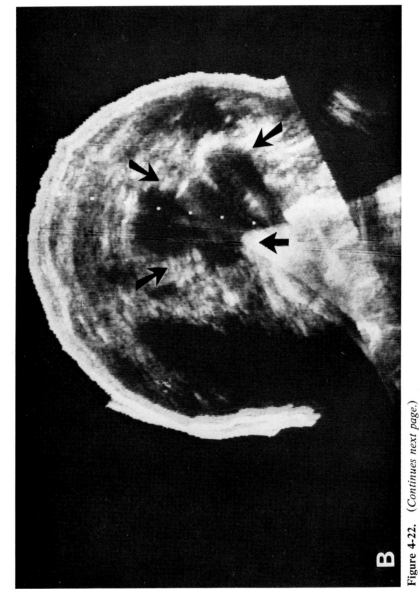

B

Figure 4-22. *(Continues next page.)*

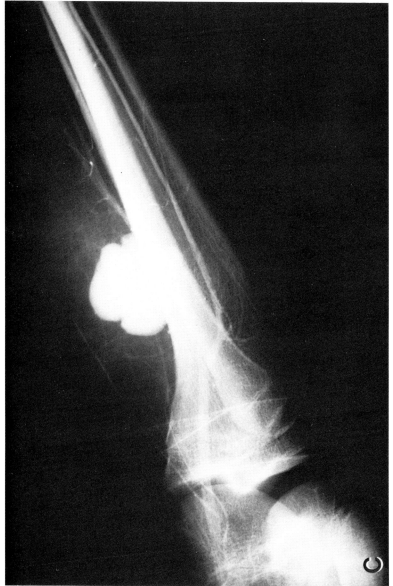

Figure 4-22. Longitudinal (A) and transverse (B) scans of a patient with a pseudoaneurysm (arrows) of the tibial artery. (C) Contrast angiogram confirms the presence of a pseudoaneurysm.

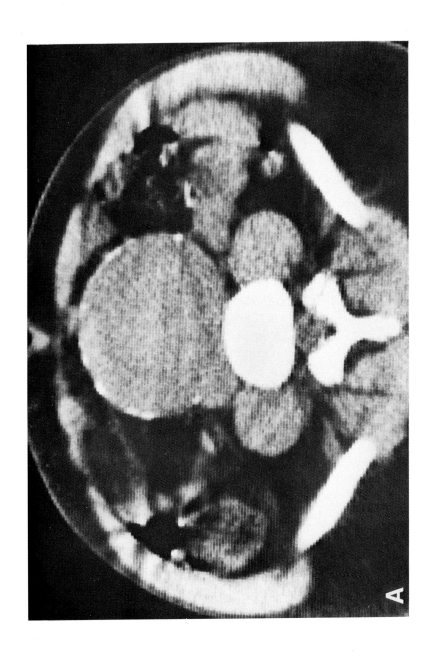

66

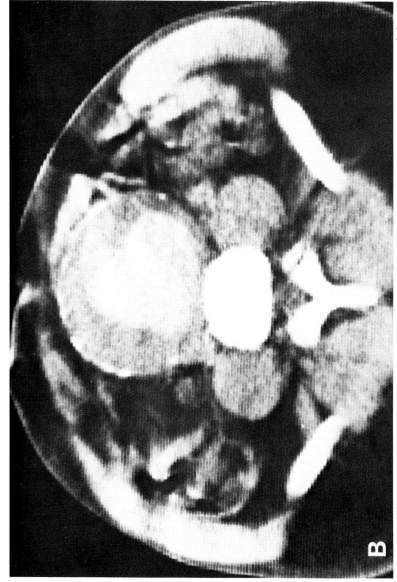

Figure 4-23. Marked enlargement of the aorta as a result of an aneurysm in the precontrast scan (A). The postcontrast scan (B) at the same level reveals a laminated mural thrombus.

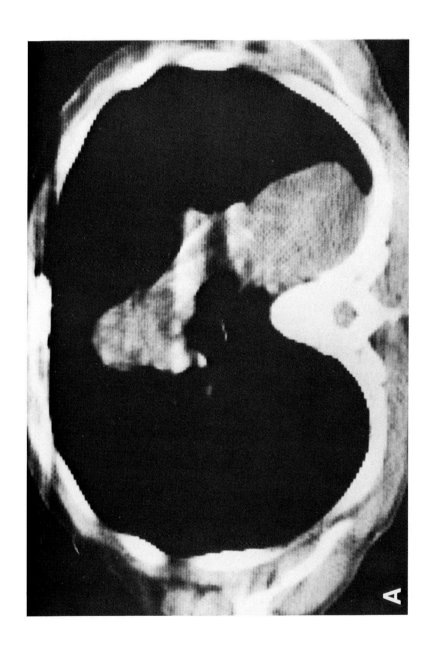

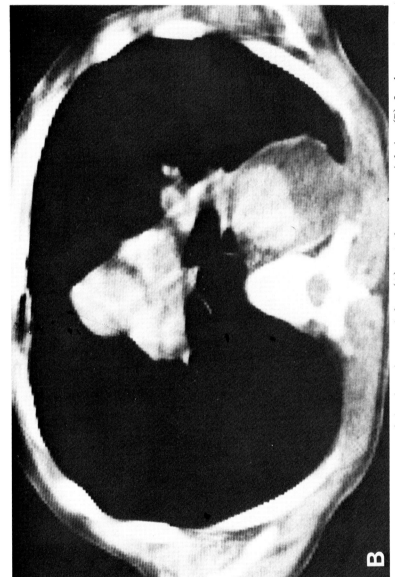

Figure 4-24. An aneurysm of the thoracic aorta before (A) and after contrast infusion (B). In the postcontrast study a moderately sized thrombus is evident.

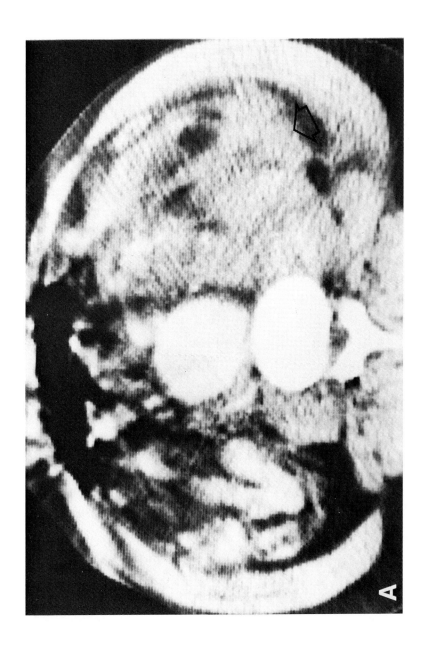

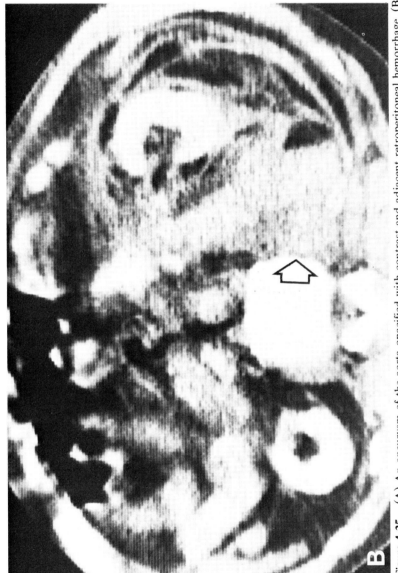

Figure 4-25. (A) An aneurysm of the aorta opacified with contrast and adjacent retroperitoneal hemorrhage. (B) Same patient, scan at renal level.

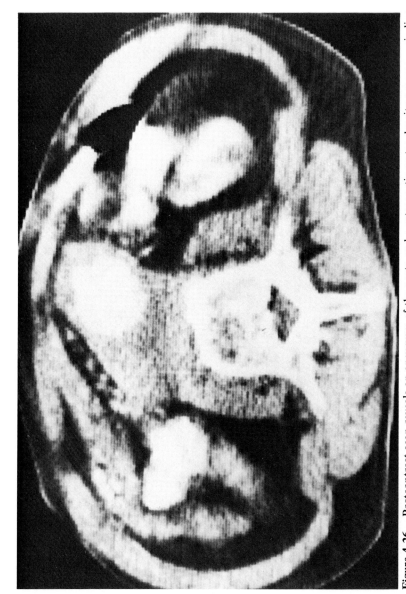

Figure 4-26. Postcontrast scan reveals an aneurysm of the aorta and a retroaortic water density process encircling the aorta. Surgery revealed periaortic metastatic lymphadenopathy.

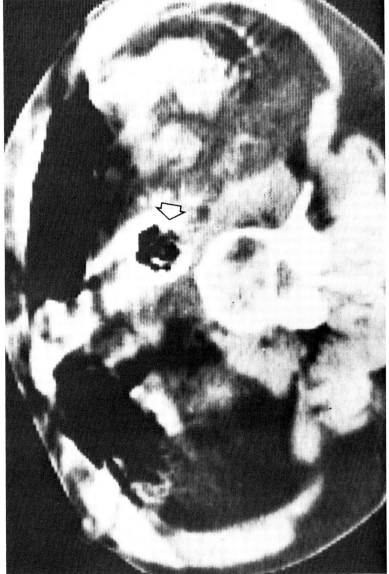

Figure 4-27. Air in the lumen of the aorta. Surgery confirmed a gas-producing infection of the thrombosed aorta.

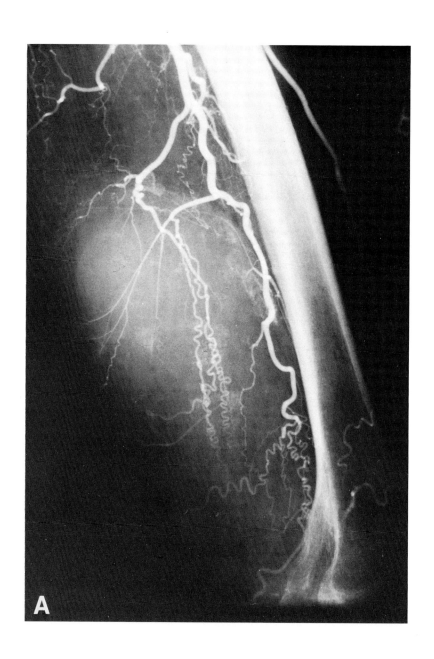

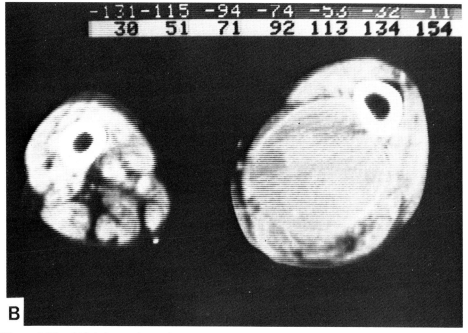

Figure 4-28. (A) A femoral arteriogram reveals occlusion of the superficial femoral artery and a mass in the thigh. (B) A postcontrast scan reveals faint opacification of the interior with a well-defined wall. Surgery revealed a pseudoaneurysm with clots inside. [Courtesy Dr S. Chandramouli, Northwest Community Hospital, Arlington Heights, Ill.]

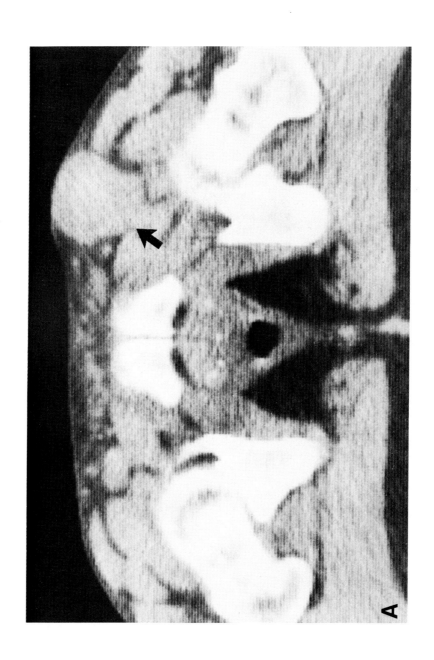

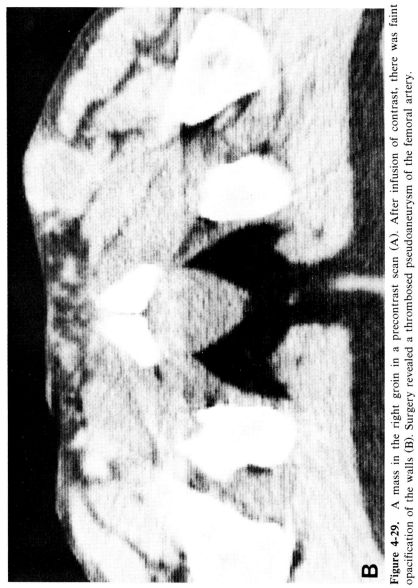

Figure 4-29. A mass in the right groin in a precontrast scan (A). After infusion of contrast, there was faint opacification of the walls (B). Surgery revealed a thrombosed pseudoaneurysm of the femoral artery.

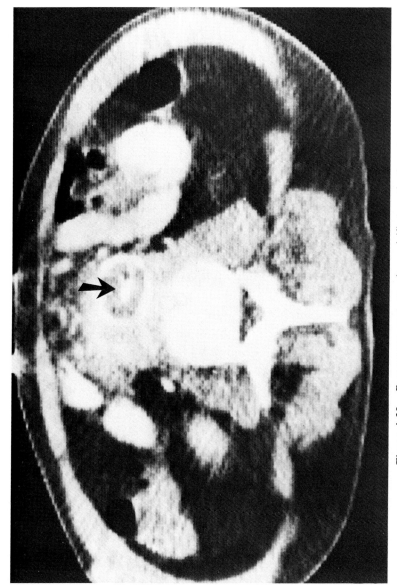

Figure 4-30. Precontrast scan reveals a calcified aortic thrombus.

of the symphysis pubis. Routine precontrast and postcontrast scans will not only demonstrate the vascular pathology better, but will also yield a better insight into the adjacent nonvascular processes.

REFERENCES

1. Leopold GN: Ultrasonic abdominal aortography. Radiology 9689, 1970
2. Winsberg F, Cole-Beuglet C, Mulder DS: Continuous ultrasound "B" scanning of abdominal aortic aneurysms. AJR 121:626, 1974
3. Wheeler WE, Beachley MC, Ranniger K: Angiography and ultrasonography: A comparative study of abdominal aortic aneurysms. AJR 126:95, 1976
4. Hirsch JH, Thiele BL, Carter SS, et al: Aortic and lower extremity arterial aneurysms. J Clin Ultrasound 9:29–31, 1981
5. Silver TM, Washburn RL, Stanley JC, et al: Gray scale ultrasound evaluation of popliteal artery aneurysms. AJR 129:1003–1006, 1977
6. Neiman HL, Lao JST, Silver TM: Gray-scale ultrasound diagnosis of peripheral arterial aneurysms. Radiology 130:413–416, 1979
7. Gooding GA, Effeney DJ: Ultrasound of femoral artery aneurysms. AJR 134:477–480, 1980
8. Nusbaum JW, Freimanis AK, Thomford NR: Echography in the diagnosis of abdominal aortic aneurysms. Arch Surg 102:385–388, 1971
9. Brewsters DC, Darling C, Rainer JK: Assessment of abdominal aortic aneurysms size. Circulation 56:164–169, 1977
10. Athey PA, Jamez L: Lateral decubitus position for demonstration of the aortic bifurcation. J Clin Ultrasound 7:154–155, 1979
11. Isikoff MB, Hill MC: Sonography of the renal arteries: Left lateral decubitus position. AJR 134:1177–1179, 1980
12. Gooding GA, Herzog KA, Hedgcock MW, et al: B-mode ultrasonography of prosthetic vascular grafts. Radiology 127:763–766, 1978
13. Wolson AH, Kaupp HA, McDonald K: Ultrasound of arterial graft surgery complications. AJR 133:869–875, 1979
14. Wyachulis AR, Spittell JA, Wallace RB: Popliteal aneurysms. Surgery 68:942–952, 1970
15. Meyers MA: Radiology of the Abdomen: Normal and Pathological Anatomy. New York, Springer Verlag, 1976
16. Whalen JP: Radiology of the Abdomen: Anatomic Basis. Philadelphia, Lea & Febiger, 1976

17. Axelbaum SP, Schellinger D, Gomes MN: Computed tomographic evaluation of aortic aneurysms. AJR 127:75–78, 1976
18. Gomes MN: ACTA scanning in the diagnosis of abdominal aortic aneurysms. Comput Tomogr 1:51–61, 1977
19. Axelbaum SP, Schellinger D, Gomes MN, et al: Computed tomographic evaluation of aortic aneurysms. AJR 127:75–78, 1976
20. Gomes MH, Hakkal HG, Schellinger D: Ultrasonography and CT scanning: A comparative study of abdominal aortic aneurysm. J Comput Assist Tomogr 2:99–109, 1978
21. Tasaka MK: CT patterns of mural thrombus in aortic aneurysms. J Comput Assist Tomogr 4:840–842, 1980
22. Sanders JH, Malave S, Neiman HL, et al: Thoracic aortic imaging without angiography. Arch Surg 114:1326–1329, 1979
23. Sandler CM, Jackson H, Kaminski RI: Right perirenal hematoma secondary to a leaking abdominal aortic aneurysm. J Comput Assist Tomogr 5:264–266, 1981
24. Graham AL, Najaffi H, Dye WS, et al: Ruptured abdominal aortic aneurysm. Arch Surg 97:1024–1031, 1968
25. Lippey ER, Deburgh M: Concurrent extraperitoneal and intracaval rupture of an abdominal aortic aneurysm. Med J Aust 1:517–518, 1978
26. Jackson RS, Cremin BJ: Angiographic demonstration of GI bleeding due to aorto-duodenal fistula. Br J Radiol 49:966–967, 1976
27. Sagel SS, Siegel MJ, Stanley RJ, et al: Detection of retroperitoneal hemmorhage by CT. AJR 129:403–407, 1977
28. Crisler C, Bahnson HT: Aneurysms of the aorta in current problems in surgery. Chicago, Yearbook of Surgery, Dec. 1972
29. Dolinskas CA, Solman N: CT of intracerebral hematomas. AJR 129:681–688, 1977
30. Suchato C, Diedrich L: Indications of dissecting aneurysm on noncontrast CT. J Comput Assist Tomogr 4:115–116, 1980
31. Schmitz LR, Jeffrey RB, Palubinskas AJ, et al: CT demonstration of septic thrombosis of inferior vena cava. J Comput Assist Tomogr 5:259–261, 1981

Siddalingappa Srikantaswamy

5
Contrast Arteriography

After the discovery of translumbar aortography by dos Santos et al. in 1929,[1] a major advance in diagnostic radiology came in 1953, with the development of percutaneous angiography by Seldinger.[2]

PREPARATION BEFORE ANGIOGRAPHY

After a detailed explanation of the procedure and its possible complications has been given to the patient, informed consent is obtained. At this time, recognition of the patient's clinical status, bleeding diathesis, and allergic history, if any, will enable the radiologist to modify the procedure and to select the best site of entry. Possible sites of entry include the femoral artery and vein at the groin, the axillary artery at the axilla, the brachial artery above the antecubital fossa, and the aorta via the translumbar route.

FEMORAL ARTERY ANGIOGRAPHY

The femoral artery at the groin can be punctured in a retrograde or an antegrade fashion. In the majority of patients, a fluoroscope can be used to locate the medial portion of the femoral head and the arterial puncture after the leg has been externally rotated and abducted. Such an approach is crucial when dealing with a nonpulsatile but patent artery, in ipsilateral angioplasty, in obese individuals, and in individuals with a pendulous abdomen. Fluoroscopic control will also help to avoid accidental punctures of the deep femoral artery or the external iliac artery. It will also facilitate effective manual compression of the artery after the procedure. If there is a significant amount of subcutaneous scar tissue at the puncture site or if lymphadenopathy is present, the contralateral side should be used, if possible. Undue concern over puncturing a graft at the groin is unnecessary. When faced with such a situation, inserting the guide wire while withdrawing the catheter will facilitate the removal of an intact catheter.

Retrograde punctures are done through a small skin incision about 2 cm below the midinguinal point with the limb externally rotated and abducted. Antegrade puncture is vital for ipsilateral femoropopliteal angioplasty, for better opacification of the pedal vessels, and for neoplastic circulations. The common femoral artery is punctured through the skin incision about 1.5 cm cephalad to the incision. A slight medial inclination of the caudally pointed needle allows the guide wire to be inserted into the superficial femoral artery rather than into the deep femoral artery. Antegrade punctures may prove to be very difficult in very obese persons or in patients in whom the bifurcation of the common femoral artery is high. In such situations, retrograde puncture of the contralateral femoral artery should be undertaken (Fig. 5-1).

Femoral Artery Puncture Technique

After thorough preoperative and aseptic preparation of the groin and the injection of local anesthetic, a small skin incision is made approximately 2 cm below the midinguinal point. The properly fixed femoral artery is punctured with a short, beveled, thin-walled 16-gauge needle with a Teflon sleeve. Slow withdrawal of the needle from the transfixed artery results in a pulsatile but continuous stream of blood. Advancing the sheath further while retrieving the needle provides additional security and avoids subintimal injections.

A 0.035-inch or 0.038-inch J guide wire is advanced through the sheath into the lower abdominal aorta. The sheath is then withdrawn and a 5F or 6F pigtail catheter

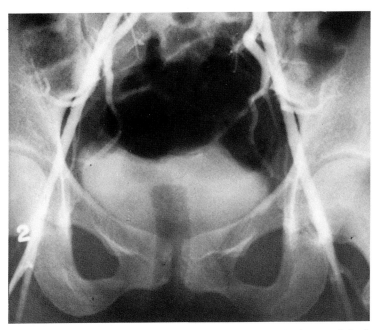

Figure 5-1. The relationship of the common femoral arteries to the heads of the femurs. The markers 1 and 2 represent skin incisions.

or a straight short catheter of the same dimensions with multiple side holes is inserted over the guide. The tip of the catheter is usually positioned about 3 to 4 inches above the aortic bifurcation. The tip can also be placed at variable levels in the thoracic or abdominal aorta, depending upon clinical needs. After the guide wire is removed, the catheter is flushed with normal saline to ensure patency. When a pigtail catheter is used, the loop should be reformed in the aorta to avoid selective injections into the lumbar artery or other major arteries. Direct connection of the catheter to the injector with no intervening stopcock insures the delivery of the contrast medium into the aorta with no external leakage near the hub of the catheter. Diluted contrast medium (60 ml of contrast plus 20 ml of saline) is then injected at the rate of 10 to 12 ml/ sec until a total of 80 ml is reached. Films of both lower extremities are made during intermittent cephalad movement of the table top while a continuous exposure rate of 1 frame/sec is maintained. Three exposures each are obtained of three areas: the lower abdomen to the groin, the groin to the knee, and the knee to the ankle. A certain amount of overlap is desirable to maintain continuity. After satisfactory films are obtained, the catheter is removed and digital compression is applied at the puncture site until the bleeding is completely controlled. The extremity is then immobilized for at least 3 to 4 hours.

Satisfactory films with uniform radiographic density can be obtained by using wedge filters. Reinjection may be needed occasionally in obese individuals or in certain situations where the velocities of flow vary. Biplane arteriography is indicated when the conventional projection does not demonstrate the lesion satisfactorily. For demonstration of the origin of the deep femoral artery, an ipsilateral anterior oblique projection may be crucial in the majority of cases, or occasionally an ipsilateral posterior oblique projection may be needed if the origin of the artery is medial.[3]

Pseudo-obstructions of an artery (e.g., anterior tibial[4,5]) may need prolonged filming with the extremity in a neutral position.

Lidocaine mixed with the contrast medium to alleviate pain may yield variable results.[6–8] If used in vessels in the upper extremities, regurgitation of the drug into the cerebral circulation may cause undesirable side effects.[9] Priscoline® (CIBA) is beneficial in relieving spasm or for better demonstration of the pedal vessels or neoplastic vasculature. Usually 25 mg of priscoline® (CIBA) is injected through the catheter 25 seconds before the injection of the contrast medium.

AXILLARY ARTERY ANGIOGRAPHY

Axillary artery puncture is undertaken when there is thrombosis of the aorta or femoral artery. Axillary artery catheterization has a higher incidence of complications, such as thrombosis, hematoma, and the secondary effects of such on the adjacent nerve bundles. Plaque dislodgement and subsequent cerebral embolization may make the clinical situation catastrophic. The left axillary artery is the route of choice for abdominal and thoracic aortic injections.

After the usual aseptic precautions and injection of local anesthetic, the arterial puncture is aimed at a point just below the axillary pectoral fold. During the puncture, the patient positions his or her palm under the head. During the injection of the J guide wire, constant fluoroscopic monitoring is vital to avoid inadvertently passing the guide wire into the branches of the subclavian or axillary artery or into the left ventricle. In the case of an ectatic aorta, a certain degree of manipulation is essential to direct the guide wire into the thoracic rather than the ascending aorta. A pigtail catheter (6F) is then advanced over the guide wire to the desired level in the abdominal aorta. The amount and rate of contrast medium injected would be similar to that for the femoral route. If aortic thrombosis is suspected, upper abdominal films are also essential. In cases of aortic thrombosis, an injection lower in the thoracic aorta may be done to opacify the femoral arteries via the intercostal collateral route.[10] Such a technique, however, exposes the spinal cord to excessive perfusion of contrast. In some instances, even a chronically thrombosed femoral artery can be punctured to inject contrast medium to better demonstrate the distal vessel (Fig. 5-2).

BRACHIAL ARTERY ANGIOGRAPHY

The brachial artery is punctured about 2 cm above the antecubital crease. Since catheterization has a higher incidence of thrombosis, only a Teflon sheath is inserted to inject the contrast medium.

After proper placement of the sheath in the artery, a total of 45 ml of contrast medium is injected over 3 seconds to opacify the subclavian and axillary systems. Films are obtained at the rate of 2/sec for 3 seconds and then 1/sec for 4 seconds. To visualize the brachial artery and its branches in the forearm, a total of 20 ml of contrast medium is injected over 4 seconds and 2 films per second for 4 seconds and 1 film per second for 3 seconds are obtained. Filming for an additional 3 to 4 seconds is needed to visualize the palmar arcade. Digital vessel opacification can be enhanced by injecting 25 mg of prescoline® (CIBA) through the catheter.[11] In individuals with Reynaud's disease,[12] better visualization of the palmar arch can be obtained by using heating pads at 33°C.

If the brachial artery cannot be punctured, then a simple curved catheter can be inserted through the femoral artery into the axillary artery. If such an approach is used, it should be kept in mind that the brachial and radial arteries sometimes have unusual proximal origins; this will help to avoid errors in interpretation (Fig. 5-3).

TRANSLUMBAR AORTOGRAPHY

The credit for inventing translumbar aortography goes to dos Santos et al.[1] This has been a very valuable procedure that yields vital information, especially when there are occlusions of the femoral arteries or aortic thrombosis.

Before translumbar aortography is used, routine ultrasonography can be used to demonstrate the presence or absence of aortic aneurysms or thrombosis, and the puncture site can be modified or another route selected. If ultrasonography is not available, then a plain abdominal film will yield some information on aortic calcifications, if present, or vertebral column abnormalities, if any. It is extremely important to obtain information about the normal coagulation profile of the patient.

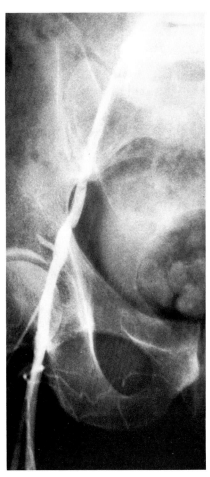

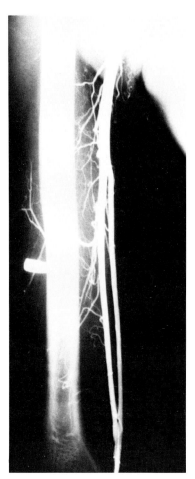

Figure 5-2. Opacification of a nonpulsatile thrombosed iliac artery in a patient who also had aortic thrombosis.

Figure 5-3. High bifurcation of the brachial artery.

Technique of Translumbar Aortography

With the patient in a prone position, the left paravertebral area at the level of the flank is prepared. The puncture site is selected at a level in between the second and third lumbar vertebral bodies and 4 inches lateral to and left of the midline. After injection of local anesthetic at the puncture site, an 8-inch 17-gauge needle is inserted through the paravertebral muscle until it strikes the anterolateral border of the lumbar vertebral body. Once the vertebral body can be felt with the needle tip, the needle is slightly withdrawn and deflected laterally to change the angle. The needle is advanced further along the side of the vertebral body until it reaches the aortic wall. Pulsations can be felt when the needle tip is in contact with the aortic wall. With short, gentle but firm thrust, the aortic wall is punctured. Once the needle is in the lumen, a pulsatile flow of blood will be noted. A test injection is then made with a small amount of contrast. This will avoid selective injections into aortic branches or subintimal injections. The needle is flushed with normal saline to ensure patency. A total of 50 ml of contrast medium over 4 seconds will satisfactorily opacify the distal vessels of the extremities along with the pelvic vessels. The filming technique is the same as that used in lower extremity arteriography. A long 19-gauge needle with a Teflon sheath can also be used to inject the contrast medium; this sheath can be inserted further in the aorta with the assistance of a J wire. A sheath provides additional security, avoids subintimal injections, and provides flexibility.

The complications of translumbar aortography are usually periaortic hematomas of variable sizes or subintimal injection of the contrast medium. Periaortic hematomas usually do not pose major problems. Subintimal injections can be avoided by using fluoroscopic control before injection of the final bolus (Fig. 5-4).

DIGITAL SUBTRACTION ANGIOGRAPHY

With the advent of sophisticated computerized techniques, intravenous aortography has regained some of its former popularity.[13] The iodine signal is logarithmically amplified, isolated by subtraction, and enhanced. Unlimited numbers of image subtractions can be obtained through electronic processing and at the same time lower levels of contrast can be used.[14–21] This new technique with certain improvements has the ability to replace many catheter angiograms, which have a higher morbidity. An added advantage of this method is that the examination can be conducted on an outpatient basis.

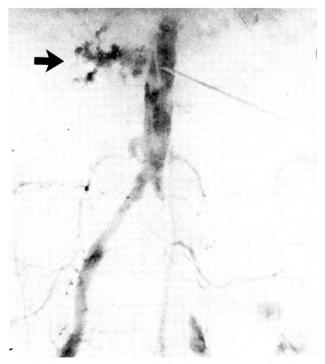

Figure 5-4. A translumbar aortogram reveals incidental extravasation (arrow) at the aortic puncture site. Also note the atherosclerotic occlusion of the left common iliac artery.

ARTERIAL ANATOMY OF THE UPPER EXTREMITIES

The subclavian artery[22,23] on the right side, which is usually a branch of the innominate artery, continues as the axillary artery at the outer border of the first rib. On the left side, the subclavian artery arises directly from the arch of the aorta. The subclavian artery on either side gives off important branches: the vertebral, internal thoracic, thyrocervical, costocervical, and dorsal scapular arteries (Fig. 5-5).

The axillary artery, which is the continuation of the subclavian artery, terminates as the brachial artery after giving rise to thoracic, scapular, and circumflex branches. The brachial artery, which is the continuation of the axillary artery, divides into the radial and ulnar arteries. The radial artery terminates in the palm by forming the deep palmar arch with the union of a deep palmar branch of the ulnar artery. The ulnar artery ends its journey in the palm by forming the superficial palmar arch, which, in turn, supplies the hand and digits. Variations of the palmar arterial patterns are not unusual.[24] Variations of the upper extremity arteries, such as direct branching of the axillary artery into the radial and ulnar arteries,[25,26] a high bifurcation of the brachial artery, or even absence of the radial artery, occasionally can be seen.[27] Incomplete palmar arches may be seen in a significant number of normal individuals.[28]

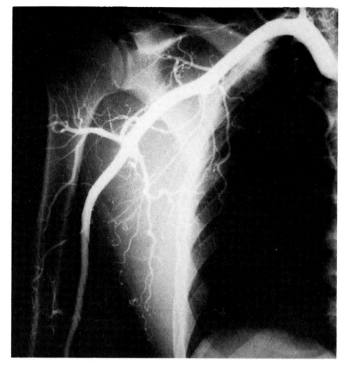

Figure 5-5.   The normal axillary artery and its branches.

ARTERIAL ANATOMY OF THE LOWER EXTREMITIES

The abdominal aorta,[22,23] after giving rise to its last branch, the middle sacral artery, bifurcates into the common iliac trunks at about the level of the fourth lumbar vertebra. The middle sacral artery usually gives rise to the paired fifth lumbar arteries. The remaining four paired lumbar arteries arise from the abdominal aorta. The common iliac trunks in turn divide into the internal and external iliac arteries in the pelvis (Fig. 5-6).

The internal iliac artery supplies the pelvic viscera and the buttocks through its anterior and posterior branches, respectively. The anterior branches are the obturator, the internal pudendal, the inferior gluteal, the middle hemorroidal, the uterine, and the vesicular arteries. The posterior branches are the iliolumbar, the lateral sacral, and the superior gluteal arteries. In the event of occlusion of the iliac arterial system, the gluteal, the iliolumbar, and the middle sacral arteries act as good collateral routes. The middle hemorroidal artery is a good collateral route when there is occlusion of the lower abdominal aorta.

The common femoral artery is a continuation of the external iliac artery at the midinguinal point. At this level it usually gives rise to superficial branches and also the deep femoral artery. The common femoral artery then continues as the popliteal artery around the adductor canal and eventually trifurcates into the posterior tibial, the peroneal, and the anterior tibial arteries (Figs. 5-7, 5-8).

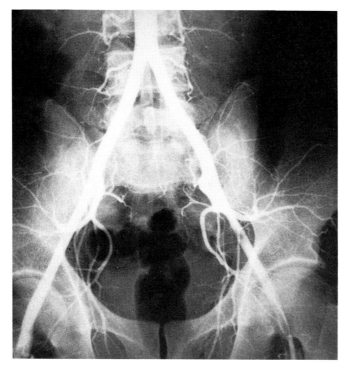

Figure 5-6. The common iliac arteries and their continuation as the common femoral arteries.

The deep femoral artery gives rise to muscular branches, perforating arteries, and circumflex femoral branches, which act as good collaterals in the event of occlusion of the common femoral artery. The deep femoral artery is a good collateral route when there is occlusion of the superior femoral artery. Variations of the arteries of the lower extremities may include absence of the iliac arteries,[29] high bifurcation of the popliteal artery, or absence of the branches of the popliteal artery[30,31] (Fig. 5-9).

COMPLICATIONS OF ANGIOGRAPHY

Angiographic complications can be caused by the contrast medium,[33-37] the angiographic equipment, or the local anesthetic.[38]

Contrast Medium

The adverse effects caused by intravascular contrast medium[33,39] can be attributed to vagal reactions,[40-43] the liberation of histamines,[44-47] or hyperosmolarity.[48-65] Vagal reactions can be either "vagovagal" or "vasovagal." Vagovagal reactions are the result of the liberation of acetylcholine. They are characterized by apnea, pallor, loss of consciousness, bradycardia, and hypotension. Cardiac standstill and death could occur in advanced cases.[33,39] Vasovagal reactions are caused by the loss of vasomotor tone and are characterized by tachycardia and hypotension. Irreversible reactions can result from these vagal reactions if immediate action is not taken.[40]

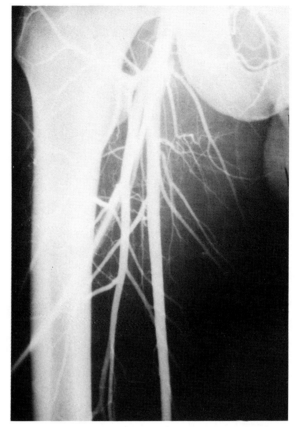

Figure 5-7. The common femoral artery and its bifurcation into the deep femoral and superficial femoral arteries.

Histamine liberation can cause angioneurotic edema,[33] bronchoconstriction, laryngospasm, urticaria, hypotension, and flushing.

Hyperosmolarity induced by contrast medium depends on the type and concentration of the contrast medium used. The osmolarity of the contrast media currently available varies from 1200 mOsm/l to 1600 mOsm/l. The effects of such hyperosmolarity on the body as a whole are innumerable. Some effects on the blood[48-57] are crenation, agglutination, sludging, rouleaux formation, alteration of coagulation,[63] capillary thrombosis, and microembolism.

Effects on the heart include an increase in cardiac load, resulting in increased pulmonary capillary venous pressure and climaxing in moderate to severe pulmonary edema.[58-62,64,65]

Pulmonary effects are acute pulmonary hypertension and acute cor pulmonale and death.[58]

Effects on the nervous system[66-69] include tetraplegia, paraplegia, hemiplegia or paresis, transient blindness, and seizures. The larger the amounts of hypertonic contrast injected, closer to the heart, the greater are the frequency and magnitude of such

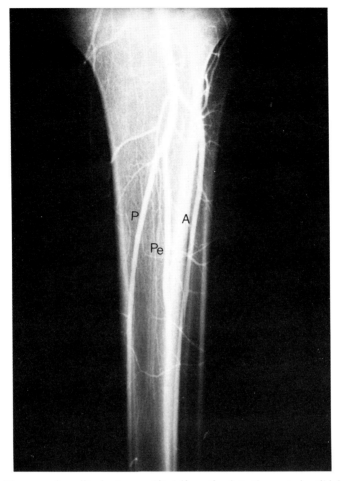

Figure 5-8. The normal popliteal artery and its trifurcation into the posterior tibial (P), peroneal (Pe) and anterior tibial (A) arteries.

reactions. The frequency of neurologic complications increases if there is decreased velocity of flow, such as is seen in aortic thrombosis or in arteria dolicho et magna. Such a relative stasis in turn causes delayed washout of the contrast medium from the spinal radiculomedullary arteries.[66-69]

Renal complications[70] are caused by the use of excessive amounts of contrast medium. This is complicated by overzealous dehydration, resulting in oliguria in individuals with limited renal reserve. This is especially true in diabetic individuals[71] who succumb to acute renal failure with limited recovery.

Excessive amounts of undiluted contrast medium may cause venous thrombosis in normal individuals[72] and even venous gangrene[73] in individuals with associated venous thrombosis. Cutaneous complications are due to inevitable or deliberate extravasation of the contrast medium resulting in tissue damage. This is especially true

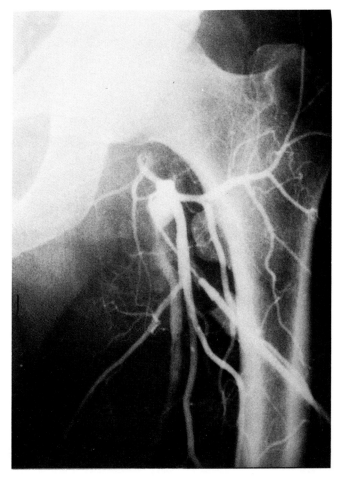

Figure 5-9. Accidental injection of contrast into the deep femoral artery.

in individuals with associated arterial insufficiency.[74,75] Cytogenetic effects of contrast media have also been experimentally documented.[76,77]

Angiographic Equipment

All catheterization procedures subject the blood, the vessels, and the tissues to variable degrees of reversible or irreversible damage. Fortunately, much of this damage is repaired by the natural healing process. Obvious clinical complications do occur when the extent of injury exceeds the healing ability of the body. These include hematomas, pseudoaneurysms, arteriovenous fistulae, thrombosis of the punctured artery,[78] atheromatous plaque dislodgement and embolization,[69,79] intimal dissection, rupture of the vessel, knotting of the catheter, broken wires or catheters in the vessel, clot formation on the catheter surface,[80,81] foreign body embolization (cotton fiber),[82] air embolization,[83–85] and rupture of angioplasty balloons.[86,87]

Local Anesthetic

The adverse effects of local anesthetic include hypersensitivity, anaphylactic reactions, convulsions, hypotensive cardiovascular collapse, and death. The local instillation of 25 mg of diphenhydramine hydrochloride (Benadryl, Parke-Davis, Morris Plains, NJ) instead of local anesthetic in allergic individuals may be beneficial.

TREATMENT OF COMPLICATIONS

Cardiac arrest should be treated by a sharp forceful blow to the anterior chest wall, external cardiac compression, and external defibrillation.[40,41,88,89] If there is no heartbeat within 3 minutes, 0.2 ml of a 1:1000 aqueous solution of epinephrine should be injected into the cardiac cavity. If there is no response to the epinephrine, 5 ml of 10-percent calcium chloride should be injected into the cardiac cavity. (Caution: Injection of either epinephrine or calcium chloride into the cardiac muscle will cause necrosis.)

The rate for external cardiac compression should be 60/min for adults and 60–90/min for infants and children. Airway restoration should be carried out and the patient should be ventilated every third or fourth cardiac compression.

Slow intravenous infusion of sodium bicarbonate, 50–150 ml (3.75 g/50 ml) can be used to combat acidosis. Hypotension should be treated with an intravenous drip of phenylephrine hydrochloride (Neo-Synephrine Hydrochloride, Winthrop Laboratories, New York, NY) (10 mg in 500 ml of normal saline) or an intravenous drip of metaraminol bitartrate (Aramine, Merck Sharp & Dohme, West Point, Penn) (5 ml in 500 ml of normal saline). Vagal reactions can be treated with IV atropine, 4 mg every minute until the pulse rate rises. Up to 2 mg may be needed.[41,84,90] Laryngeal edema can be reduced with IV epinephrine (0.3 ml of a 1:1000 aqueous solution). If this is unsuccessful, endotracheal intubation, tracheostomy, oxygen, and hydrocortisone sodium succinate (Solu-Cortef, Upjohn, Kalamazoo, MI) (100 mg IV plus oxygen) may be necessary.

Bronchospasm should be treated with a very slow IV injection of aminophylline (250 mg in 10 ml) or epinephrine (0.1–0.3 ml of a 1:1000 aqueous solution IV).

Other minor allergic reactions can be treated with Benadryl (25 mg IV), epinephrine (0.1–0.2 ml of a 1:1000 aqueous solution), or Solu-Cortef (100 mg IV).

Patients with a definite history of allergic reactions may be protected by oral administration of prednisolone (30 mg/day) and antihistamine for 2 days before and again on the day of angiography.

Proper hydration, limited amounts of contrast medium, meticulous technique, and strict postangiographic care should help to avoid many of the other complications.

DISORDERS OF THE PERIPHERAL VESSELS

Atherosclerosis

Atherosclerosis is a disseminated generalized disorder with a patchy distribution occurring as early as the fourth decade of life.[91-96] The atheromatous lesion begins in the intima and eventually affects the media. Its effects on the caliber of the vessel are

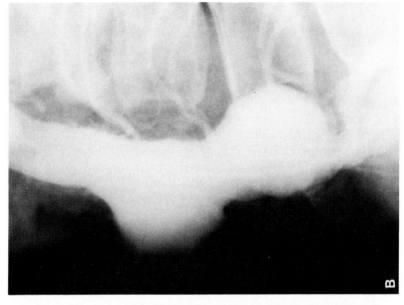

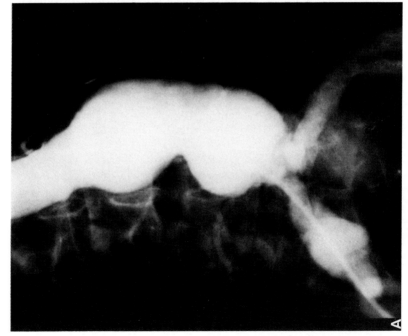

Figure 5-10. Atherosclerotic aneurysms of the aorta. (A) Anterior view. (B) Lateral view.

unpredictable. They include no change, narrowing, dilation, or occlusion. These results are due to hemorrhage into an atheroma causing narrowing or occlusion or distal atheromatous embolization.

Weakening of the media causes aneurysmal dilatation of the vessel wall. (Figs. 5-10, 5-11, 5-12) Certain segments of the vascular tree are more susceptible to the development of atheroma than others. This may be due to the repeated mechanical stress of bending or rotational movements near the joint or changes in the direction of blood flow or the nonyielding nature of the pulsating walls, e.g., the superficial femoral artery at the adductor canal or the abdominal aorta in front of the vertebral bodies).

The involved vessel usually shows a proximal progression of the disease; very rarely is the progression distal. Distal progression is more dangerous, since it may compromise the collateral vessels. The occluded vessel usually does not show evidence of recanalization or widening. Angiography, unlike autopsy, usually underestimates the extent of lesions.[97,98] It is interesting to note that conducting arteries (e.g., aorta, iliac, superficial femoral, and popliteal arteries) are extensively involved, unlike the distributing arteries. Extensive involvement of the distributing arteries is not a rarity either (Fig. 5-13).

Embolism

One of the dramatic and castrophic manifestations of atherosclerosis is embolism. Embolism is unlike thrombosis, although thrombosis, when acute, can mimic the clinical picture of embolism. Most emboli originate from the heart, but atheromatous

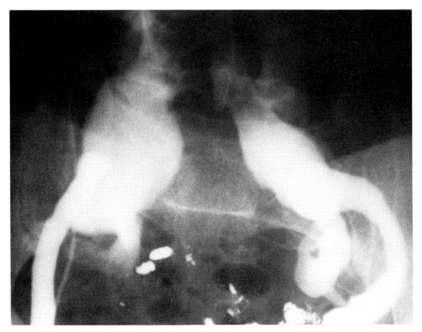

Figure 5-11. Bilateral atherosclerotic aneurysms of the iliac arteries.

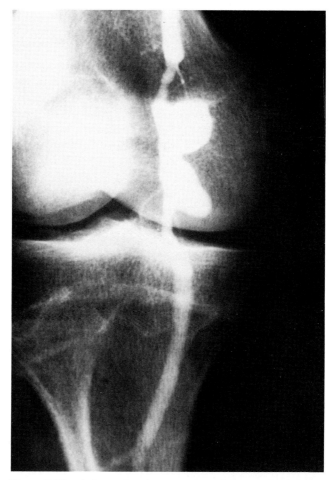

Figure 5-12. Atherosclerotic aneurysms of the popliteal artery.

great vessels are also contributors.[99-111] Emboli from tumors may be rare, but create a clinical curiosity when they do occur.[112-115] Paradoxical emboli from venous thrombi in obese individuals[116] and the case of a bullet as an embolus[117] are also interesting. Angiographic embolic agents can always dislodge and embolize into peripheral vessels[118] (Figs. 5-14–5-18).

Thrombosis

Chronic or acute thrombosis usually complicates an underlying atheromatous vessel. An increase in viscosity or platelets, or decreased perfusion pressure can set the stage for acute thrombosis of a diseased vessel.[119] Multiple lesions in the same vascular tree are common. Dominant distal lesions may mask a significant proximal lesion. The thrombosed vessel usually does not recanalize or dilate.[120]

Atherosclerotic aortic thrombosis deserves special mention. The thrombosis is usually chronic and stops below the level of the renal arteries. Associated thrombosis

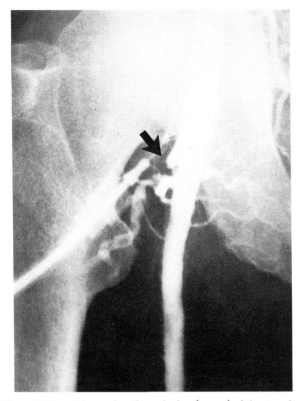

Figure 5-13. Atherosclerotic occlusion (arrow) of the deep femoral artery.

of the common iliac arteries is not unusual.[121] Occasionally aortic thrombosis is caused by repeated minimal emboli from the cardiac chambers[122] or it could be caused by proximal extension from a nonatherosclerotic disorder.[123] Rarely, of course, it may be mimic massive aortic embolization[124] when the thrombosis is acute (Fig. 5-19).

Arterial thrombosis in the lower extremities is usually caused by atherosclerosis. When there is only superficial femoral artery occlusion, collateral circulation is via the deep femoral artery. This is in contrast to femoropopliteal or popliteal occlusions. The distal circulation in diabetic individuals is very poor, since there is thrombosis of distal small vessels with centripetal progression. Other rare causes of peripheral arterial thrombosis include arteritis, thromboangiitis obliterans, radiation exposure,[125] sickle cell anemia,[126] venous thrombosis causing arterial thrombosis,[127] and ergotism[128-131] (Figs. 5-20–5-26).

Aneurysms

Aneurysmal dilatation of a vessel is the result of damage to the medial elastic layers caused by intimal atheroma. Occasionally, aneurysms can be the result of trauma, infection, or arteritis.[132-139] Fibrotic reaction induced by the aneurysm surrounds the adventitia and a puddle of blood layers it with laminated intraluminal

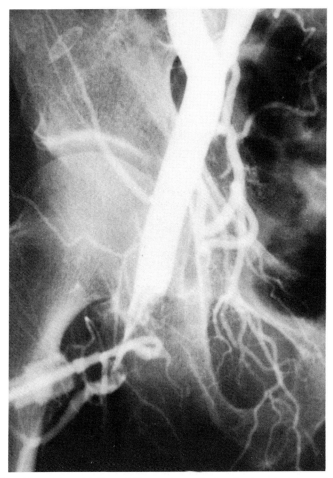

Figure 5-14. Abrupt termination of the common femoral artery because of an embolus.

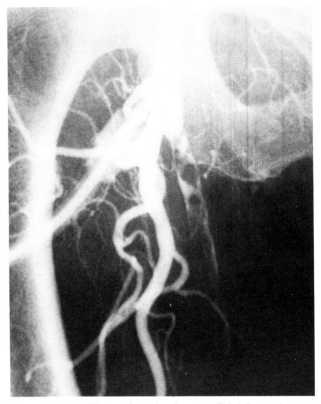

Figure 5-15. Filling defects in the superficial femoral artery because of an embolus.

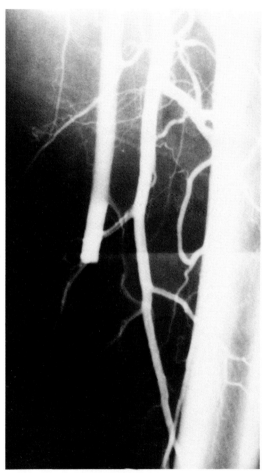

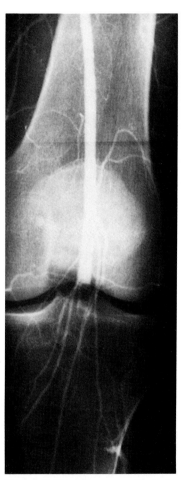

Figure 5-16. Sharp cutoff of the superficial femoral artery because of an embolus.

Figure 5-17. Sharp cutoff of the popliteal artery because of an embolus.

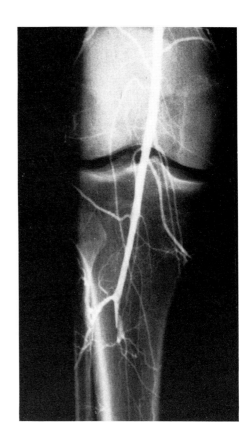

Figure 5-18. Embolic occlusion of the branches of the popliteal artery.

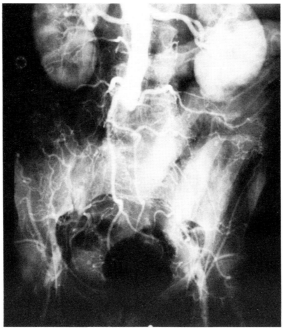

Figure 5-19. Aortic occlusion caused by aortic thrombosis.

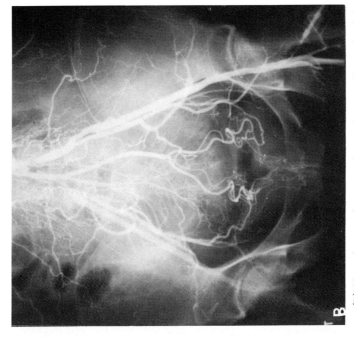

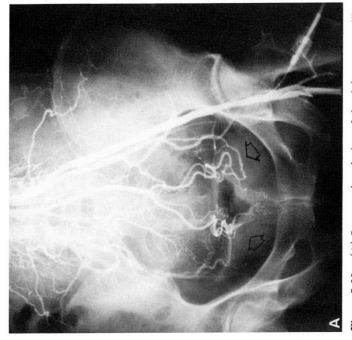

Figure 5-20. (A) Segmental occlusion of the right common iliac artery. (B) Note the prominent rectal branches opacifying the right internal iliac and external iliac arteries via the pudendal arteries.

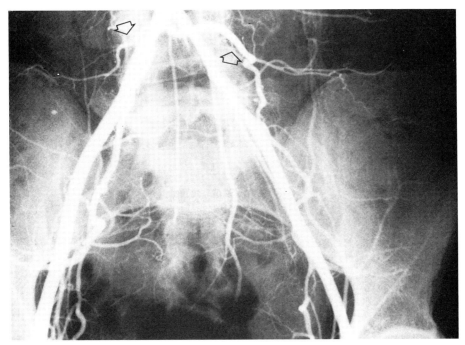

Figure 5-21. Atherosclerotic narrowing of the left common iliac artery. There is associated dilatation of the left lumbar artery caused by collateral circulation (open arrows).

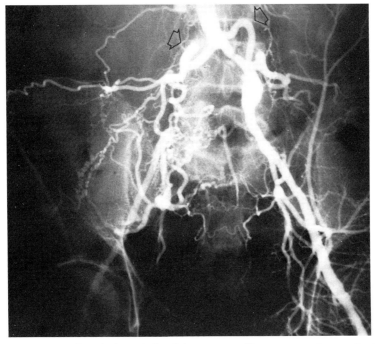

Figure 5-22. Segmental occlusion of the right common iliac artery and stenosis of the left common artery with poststenotic dilatation. Note also the dilated lumbar arteries.

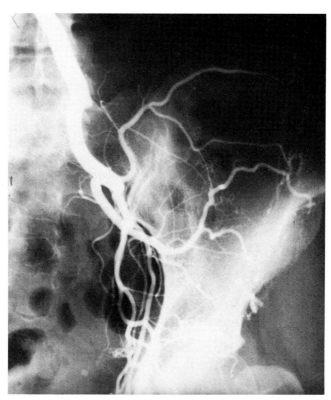

Figure 5-23. Occulsion of left external iliac artery with collaterals to the femoral artery via the gluteal arteries.

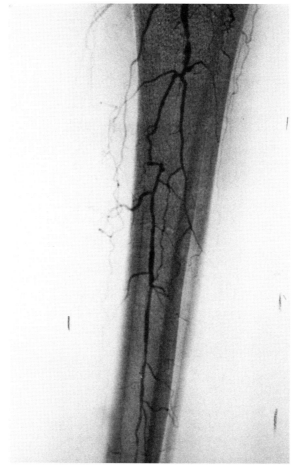

Figure 5-24. Atherosclerotic occlusions of the popliteal artery branches. Collaterals are opacifying one branch of the popliteal artery.

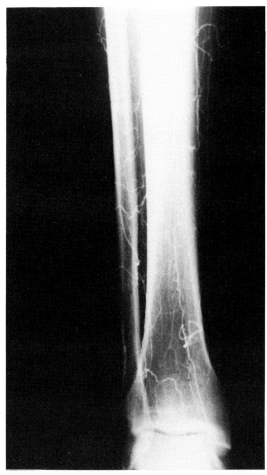

Figure 5-25. Inefficient collaterals to the calf in an individual with atherosclerotic occlusion of the popliteal trifurcation.

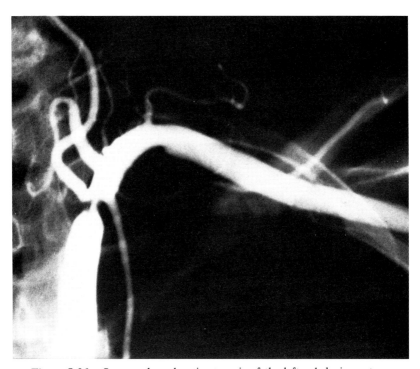

Figure 5-26. Severe atheroslerotic stenosis of the left subclavian artery.

thrombus. Constant systolic thrust and lignifaction of the thrombus cause further weakening of the already damaged wall, resulting in rupture.[140] This is especially true in atherosclerotic abdominal aortic aneurysms that are greater than 5 cm in diameter.[141,142] The effects of aneurysms on the circulation are various, such as mechanical pressure on the adjacent vessels, spontaneous rupture into the neighboring vein, distal emboli from mural thrombus, or even total thrombosis of the arterial lumen.[143-145]

Unlike syphilitic aneurysms, atherosclerotic aortic aneurysms usually occur below the level of the renal arteries.[95,146] Associated aneurysms elsewhere are not unusual.[147] There is a great threat of spontaneous rupture of an aneurysm when it attains a diameter of more than 5 cm.[141,142] When it ruptures it is usually into the retroperitoneum, and occasionally into the peritoneal cavity,[148] the duodenum,[149] the perirenal space,[150] or into the inferior vena cava.[151] (Fig. 5-27). Other miscellaneous causes of aneurysm include vascular grafts,[152,153] giant cell arteritis,[154] and a persistent primitive sciatic artery.[155-157]

Popliteal artery aneurysms need special mention. Because of their location, silent thromboembolic complications,[143-145,158] venous thrombosis,[159] or even rupture[160-163] may occur. They can be single and saccular in normotensives or fusiform and bilateral in hypertensive individuals (see Fig. 5-12).

Other aneurysms of special interest are true traumatic aneurysms either resulting from acute blunt or chronic minimal blunt trauma. The latter usually due to contusion of the arterial wall with progressive dilatation.[164-170] Mycotic aneurysms are caused by bacterial infections either by implantation or direct involvement. The end result is destruction of the elastic walls with dilatation and fatal rupture. The common sites are on the abdominal vessels, although atherosclerotic vessels in the extremities are frequent sites in the elderly[171,172] (Fig. 5-28).

Trauma

Blunt, penetrating, or osseous trauma can cause varieties of vascular damage. These include contusion, compression, subintimal or adventitial hematomas, intimal fractures, complete laceration, pseudoaneurysms, and arteriovenous fistulae.[173-176] Immediate clinical examination usually reveals the extent of vascular damage. But in some instances a latent period is not unusual, during which formation of thrombus occurs. Arteries in the vicinity of osseous structures are highly vulnerable when there is associated osseous trauma.[177,178] This is especially true of the common iliac arteries and their branches.[179,180] Some examples include the internal pudendal and obturator artery in cases of pubic fracture,[219] and the superior gluteal artery and common iliac vessels[181,182] at the sacroiliac joint. Apart from osseous traumas, even blunt traumas can cause significant damage to these vessels.[182-184] When there is a laceration or avulsion of an artery, as is usually associated with large hematomas, some of them eventually become pseudoaneurysms. (Fig. 5-29–5-33)

High velocity missiles, while traversing adjacent to an artery, can cause variable degrees of damage to the artery because of violent vibrations during passage. Such an event could result in intimal dehiscence, aneurysms, or even thrombosis. Due to the generated heat delayed complications such as hematomas, aneurysms, and arteriovenous fistulae can also occur.[185-187] (Fig. 5-34, 5-35)

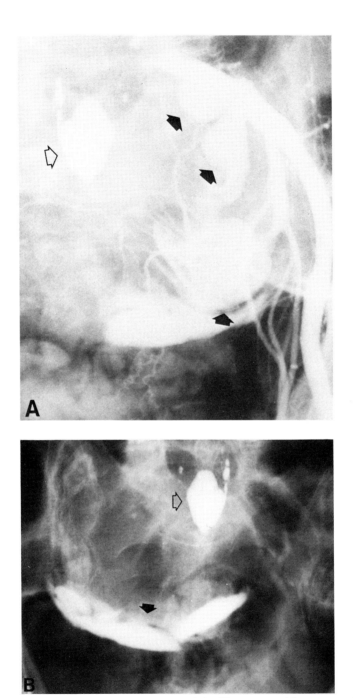

Figure 5-27. Multiple atherosclerotic aneurysms of the iliac artery with extravasation of the contrast. Note incidental Myelographic contrast (open arrow). (B) Extravasated contrast in a periaterial cavity (closed arrow).

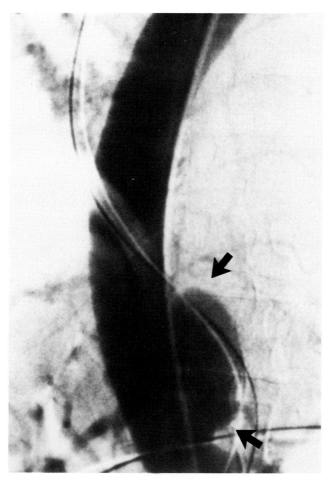

Figure 5-28. Periaortic collection of contrast (arrows) caused by a mycotic aneurysm in a drug abuser.

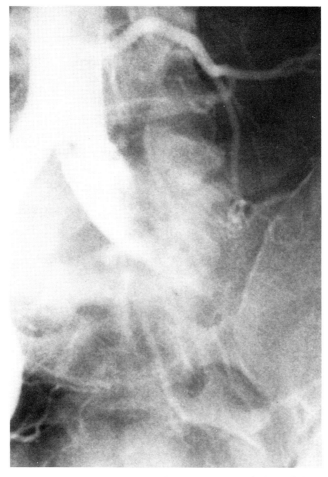

Figure 5-29. Irregular walls of the common iliac artery and occlusion of the artery caused by intimal laceration and avulsion.

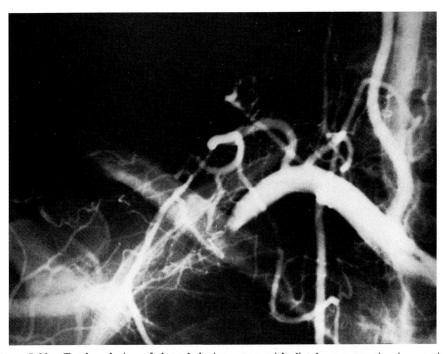

Figure 5-30. Total occlusion of the subclavian artery with distal reconstruction in a patient who received a stab wound.

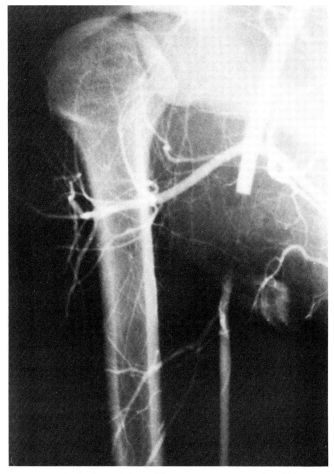

Figure 5-31. Occlusion of the axillary artery as a result of blunt trauma.

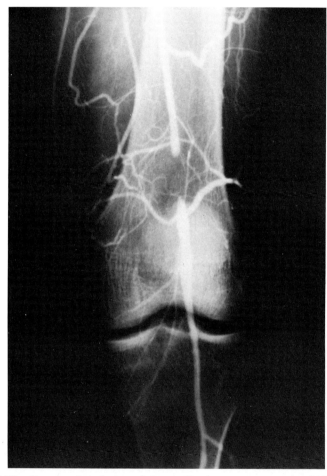

Figure 5-32. Segmental occlusion of the popliteal artery as a result of blunt trauma.

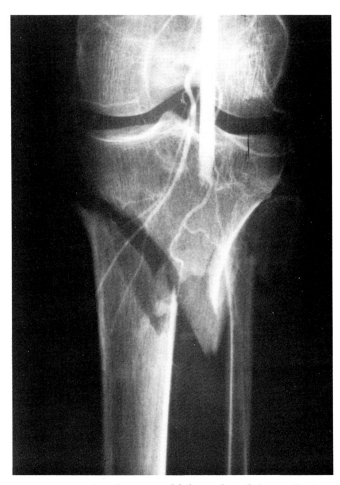

Figure 5-33. Obvious fractures with laceration of the popliteal artery.

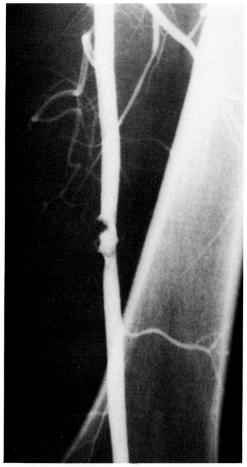

Figure 5-34. Irregularity of the superficial femoral artery caused by a missile injury resulting in subadventitial hematoma and intimal laceration.

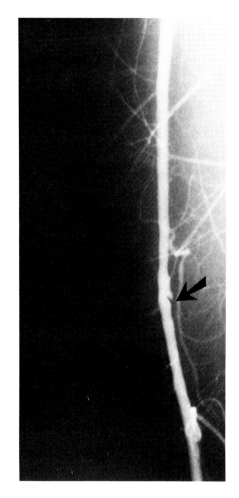

Figure 5-35. Dehiscence of the intima (arrow) of the superficial femoral artery caused by a missile injury.

Repeated minimal blunt trauma can cause intimal trauma or contusion of the vessel wall with eventual thrombosis, as seen in palmar or digital arteries.[143] Long term use of crutches can do the same to the brachial artery.[169] An angiographic catheter may itself induce arterial thrombosis due either to intimal trauma or spasm resulting in stasis and eventual thrombosis.

Pseudoaneurysm

A pseudoaneurysm is usually the end result of a penetrating trauma due to a defect in the arterial wall. They are periarterial hematomas of variable sizes; the size of the hematoma and the formation of a wall around it depends upon the coagulation mechanisms, status of blood pressure, and the type of resistance from surrounding tissues. Further expansion of such a hematoma and fatal rupture depends on the same defense mechanisms of the body. A pseudoaneurysm could also occur due to infections like salmonella, staphylococcus, enterobacteria, or tuberculosis organisms.[171,188] Post-angiographically or surgically caused pseudoaneurysms are also common. (Fig. 5-36–5-39)

Arteriovenous Fistula

Penetrating or blunt trauma is the major cause of acquired arteriovenous fistulae. Iatrogenic trauma due to surgery or diagnostic procedures may also be included in this category. Such a communication, in fact, is an engrafted parasitic "short circuit," imposed upon a normal circulation. Sudden shunting of the blood with its hemodynamic changes imposes a burden on the heart, resulting in increased cardiac output and eventual failure. Such outcome depends on its proximity of the communication to the heart, volume of blood per cardiac cycle shunted, and the length and size of the fistula.[189–191] Usually small peripheral AV fistulae produce insignificant hemodynamic changes.[190] (Fig. 5-40–5-42)

EXTRINSIC COMPRESSION

Thoracic Outlet Syndrome

The narrowing or occlusion of the subclavian artery at the thoracic outlet level is usually due to numerous structures.[192–194] Posteriorly, the artery and the vein can be compressed by the cervical rib, scalenus medius, or fibrous bands; anteriorly, by scalenus anterior, clavicle, or costoclavicular ligament. Repeated chronic pressure could cause structural changes in the vessel wall with narrowing or thrombosis and distal or proximal embolization. The only clinical manifestation in some individuals could be due to distal embolization of upper extremity vessels. Anatomic abnormality could be present with no hemodynamic changes.[195] At the axilla, pressure changes on the axillary artery can be from the pectoralis minor, the head of the humerus or the median nerve. (Fig. 5-43, 5-44)

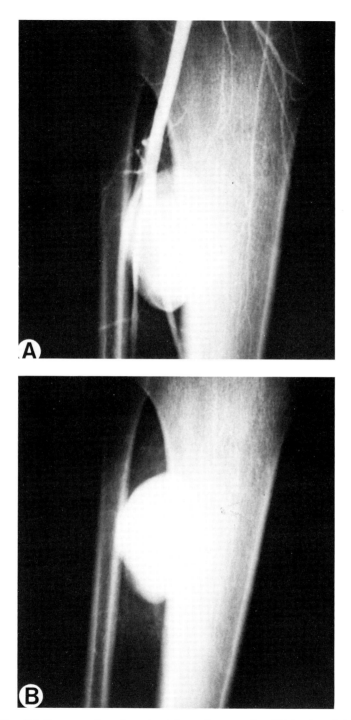

Figure 5-36. (A) Extravasation of contrast from the posterior tibial artery into a traumatic pseudoaneurysm. (B) Note persistent opacification of the pseudoaneurysm.

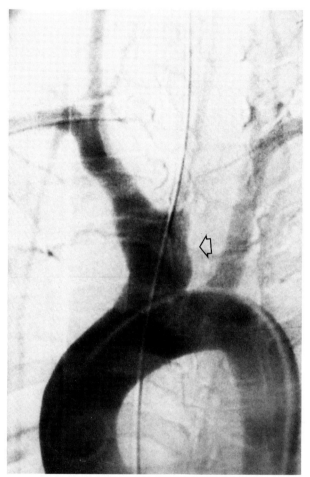

Figure 5-37. Dilatation and irregularity of the innominate artery as a result of avulsion and an associated pseudoaneusym.

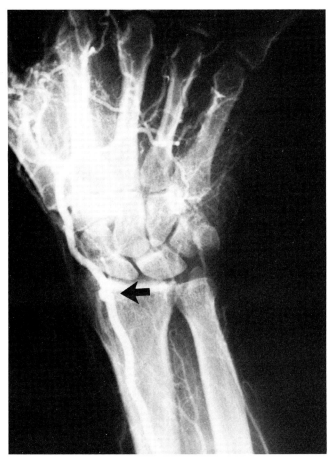

Figure 5-38. A small pseudoaneurysm (arrow) of the radial artery caused by a knife blade injury.

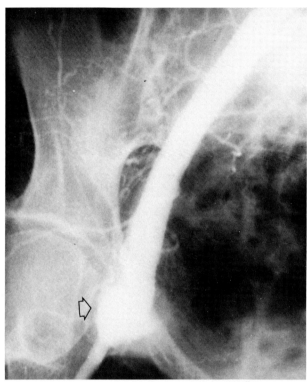

Figure 5-39. A pseudoaneurysm (arrow) at the anastomosis of a graft.

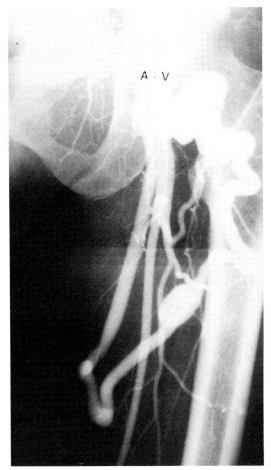

Figure 5-40. Simultaneous opacification of the femoral artery and vein caused by a traumatic arteriovenous communication (AV) at the level of medial femoral circumflex branch.

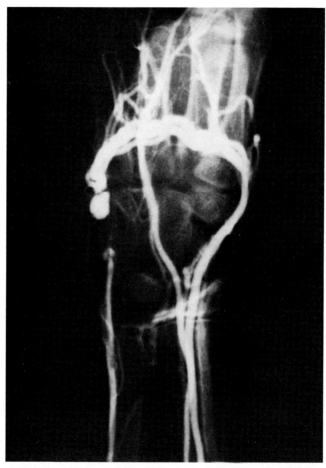

Figure 5-41. Simultaneous opacification of the artery and vein of the palmar arch because of a traumatic arteriovenous communication. Also note the occlusion of the distal ulnar artery.

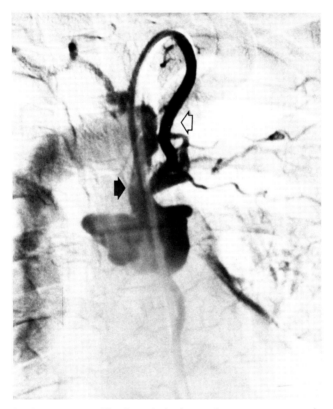

Figure 5-42. Simultaneous opacification of the internal mammary artery (open arrow) and vein (closed arrow) and the innominate vein because of a traumatic arteriovenous fistula.

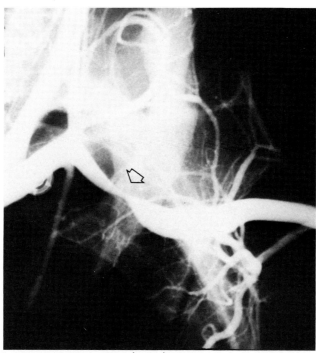

Figure 5-43. Stress-induced narrowing (arrow) of the subclavian artery caused by scalenus anticus syndrome. [Courtesy Dr S. Chandramouli, Northwest Community Hospital, Arlington Heights, Ill.]

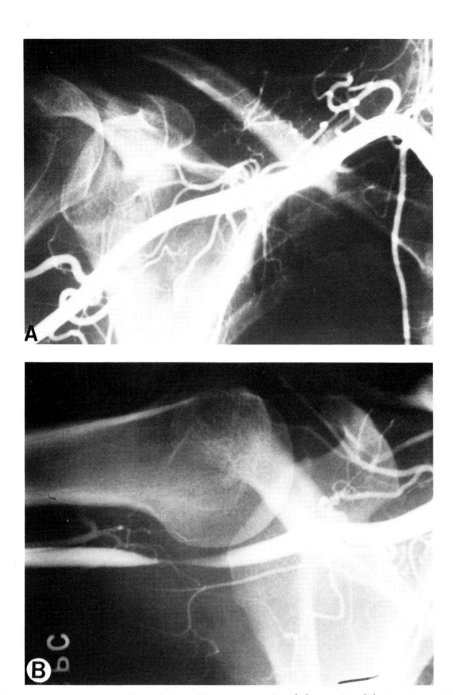

Figure 5-44. Note the caliber of the axillary artery before (A) and after (B) abduction of the arm in a patient with hyperabduction syndrome with distal transient circulatory changes. [Courtesy of Dr S. Chandramouli, Northwest Community Hospital, Arlington Heights, Ill.]

Popliteal Artery Entrapment

Entrapment of the popliteal artery by the medial head of the gastronemius muscle can cause narrowing or occlusion. This entity, presenting with claudication, can often be bilateral and is frequently seen in young individuals.[143,196,197] (Fig. 5-45) Anterior tibial compartment syndrome[198,199] is usually due to hemorrhage in the anterior tibial compartment with extrinsic compression of the patent anterior tibial artery. Delayed filming will demonstrate the patent artery and helps to modify the surgical procedure.

Miscellaneous Disorders

Medial calcific sclerosis, arteritis, fibromuscular dysplasias, and thromboangiitis obliterans also occur. They usually involve the distribution of medium and small vessels that are rich in muscle. Occasionally, diseases such as arteritis and aortitis may involve both large and medium vessels. Rare are the congenital disorders causing narrowing of the aorta[200] or femoral arteries or disorders caused by exposure of the aorta[201] or subclavian artery to radiation.[202] Mucoid cystic adventitial degeneration of the arterial wall, which is frequently seen in younger individuals, causes narrowing or occlusion. This disorder is commonly seen in the popliteal artery but occasionally in other vessels in the extremities.[203,204]

Neurofibromatous tissue in the vessel wall can cause narrowing as a result of intimal and medial fibrous proliferation.[205-207]

Medial calcific sclerosis[98] is a disorder of the medium and smaller muscular arteries without encroachment on their lumen[91] (Fig. 4-2). When the calcified vessel fractures, there is associated vascular thrombosis and associated ischemic changes.[208] Even a pseudoaneurysm caused by fracture of the wall may not be an uncommon occurrence (Fig. 4-2). Arteritis is a disease of the vascular wall with an unknown etiology. It has a patchy diffuse distribution and mostly affects young women. It is a panarteritis with intimal proliferation, thrombosis, and organization resulting in smooth obstruction or stenosis. Patchy destruction of the media may cause aneurysmal dilatation. Aortitis, Takayasu arteritis, and giant cell arteritis may be included under this disorder.[132-137] Fibromuscular dysplasia constitutes a group of nonatherosclerotic arterial lesions that have a higher incidence in women. Because of the disruption and hyperplastic changes of the intima, media, or adventitia, there is narrowing or dilatation of the involved vessel.[209] Although the renal arteries are frequently involved, the iliac,[210] femoral,[211] arteries and even the aorta are not immune (Fig. 5-46). Thromboangiitis obliterans is an inflammatory type of vascular disease usually involving the vessels of the lower extremities. Smooth narrowing and gradual obliteration of the vessels are the end results. Centripetal progression with no skipping of areas distinguishes this disease from atherosclerosis[212,213] (Fig. 5-47).

Arteria dolicho et magna[214] is the result of a loss of elastic tissue because of aging with subsequent dilatation and an increase in length of the aorta and its branches. Superimposed atherosclerosis is a frequent finding. An extremely decreased velocity of blood flow, which causes circulatory insufficiency of the distal circulation, is noteworthy. Superimposed mural thrombi with distal embolization and thrombosis of arteries makes the clinical situation worse (see Figs. 5-48, 5-49).

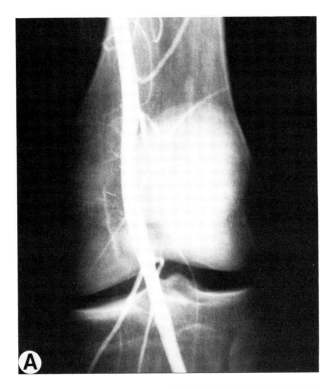

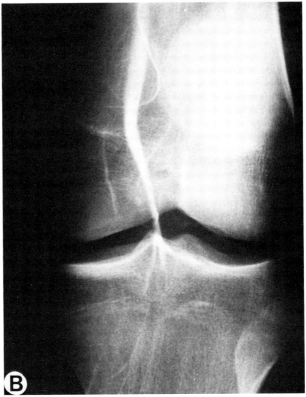

Figure 5-45. (*Continues next page.*)

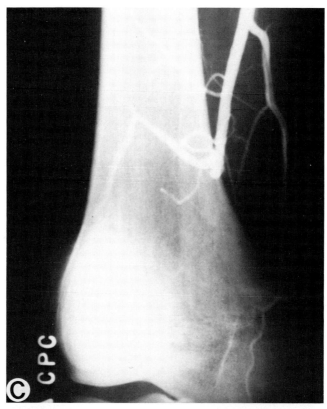

Figure 5-45. The popliteal artery before (A) and after (B) plantar flexion of the left foot. Note the complete occlusion of the right popliteal artery (C). This young individual had bilateral intermittent claudication. These findings are suggestive of popliteal artery entrapment by the gastrocnemius muscle. [Courtesy of Dr S. Chandramouli, Northwest Community Hospital, Arlington Heights, Ill.]

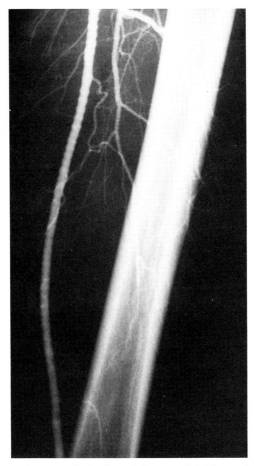

Figure 5-46. Smooth rippling of the superficial femoral artery caused by stationary waves.

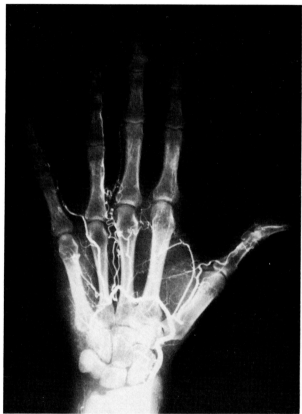

Figure 5-47. Occlusion of the digital arteries in a patient with thromboangiitis obliterans.

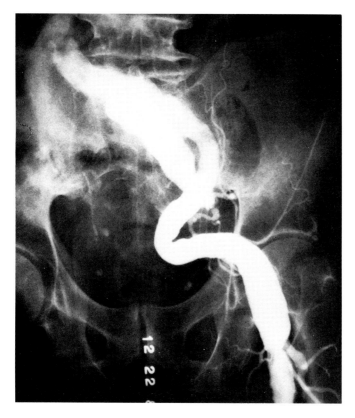

Figure 5-48. Diffuse dilatation of the iliac artery and its branches (arteria dolicho et magna).

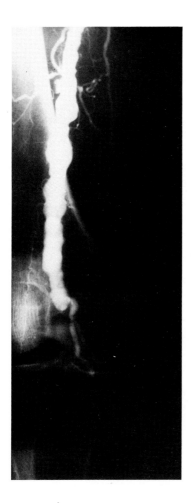

Figure 5-49. Total occlusion of the popliteal artery in a patient with arteria dolicho et magna.

REFERENCES

1. Dos Santos R, Lamas A, Perieracaldos J: L'arteriographie des membres de l'aorte et de ser branches abdominales. Soc Nat Chir Bull Med 55:587–592, 1929

2. Seldinger ST: Catheter replacement of the needle in percutaneous arteriography. Acta Radiol [Diag] 39:368–376, 1953

3. Freiman DB, Oleaga JA, Ring EJ: Angiography of the femoral bifurcation. Radiology 131:254, 1979

4. Gitlitz GF: Anterior tibial compartment syndrome. Vasc Dis 2:122–130, 1965

5. Koolpa HA, Embil W, et al: Pseudoobstruction of the anterior tibial artery. AJR 134:749–752, 1980

6. Widrich WC, Robbins AH, Goldstein SA, et al: Adjuvant intraarterial lidocaine in aortofemoral arteriography. Radiology 129:371–373, 1978

7. Eisenberg RL, Mani RL, Hedgcock MW: Pain associated with peripheral angiography: Is lidocaine effective? Radiology 127:109–111, 1978

8. Yoram-Ben Menachem: Paradoxic response to intraarterial lidocaine analgesia. AJR 130:360–361, 1978

9. Chauang VP, Widrich WC: Complications from intraarterial lidocaine in upper extremity arteriography. AJR 131:906, 1978

10. Vine HS, Sacks BA: Visualization of the distal arterial vessels in complete aortic occlusion. AJR 134:847–848, 1980

11. Jacobs JB, Hahafee WN: Use of priscoline in peripheral arteriography. Radiology 88:957–960, 1967

12. Rosch J, Antonovic R, Porter JM: The importance of temperature in angiography of the hand. Radiology 123:323–326, 1977

13. Steinberg J: Intravenous aortography. AJR 92:893–890, 1964

14. Crummy AB, Strother, CM, et al: Computerized fluoroscopy. AJR 135:1131–1140, 1980

15. Strother CM, Javid MJ: Clinical applications of computerized fluoroscopy. Radiology 136:781–783, 1980

16. Meaney TF, Weinstein MA, et al: Digital subtraction angiography. AJR 135:1153–1160, 1980

17. Reuter SR: Digital subtraction angiography (editorial). AJR 135:1316, 1980

18. Misretta CA, Crummy AB, et al: Digital angiography, a perspective. Radiology 139:273–278, 1981

19. Hillman BJ, Ovitt TW, et al: Digital video subtraction angiography of renal vascular abnormalities. Radiology 139:277–280, 1981

20. Buonocore E, Meaney TF, et al: Digital subtraction angiography of the abdominal aorta and renal arteries. Radiology 139:281–286, 1981

21. Chilocote WA, Modic MD, et al: Digital subtraction angiography of the carotid arteries. Radiology 139:287–295, 1981

22. Morris in Anson BJ (ed): Human Anatomy. New York, McGraw Hill, 1966

23. Warwick R, Williams PL (eds): Gray's Anatomy. Philadelphia, W.B. Saunders, 1973

24. Coleman SS: Arterial patterns in hand. Surg Gynecol Obstet 113:409–416, 1961

25. Huelke DF: Variation in the branches of axillary artery. Anat Rec 135:33–41, 1959

26. Sutton D: Arteriography of the upper extremities, in Abrams HL (ed): Angiography (ed 2), vol 2. Boston, Little Brown, 1971

27. Chatrapathi DN: Absence of radial artery. Indian Med Sci 18:462–465, 1964

28. Mitra SK: Terminal distribution of hepatic artery. J Anat 100:651–663, 1966

29. Doumanian AV, Frahm CJ, et al: Intermittent claudication secondary to congenital absence of iliac arteries. Arch Surg 91:604–606, 1965

30. Bardsley JL, Staple TW: Variation in the branching of the popliteal artery. Radiology 94:581–587, 1970

31. Sackler JP, Abrams RM, Berambaum ER: Congenital absence of the anterior tibial artery. Angiology 19:67–74, 1968

32. Hessel SJ: Complications of angiography. Radiology 138:273–280, 1981

33. Ansell G: Adverse reactions to contrast agent. Invest Radiol 5:374–384, 1970

34. Phillips JH, Burch GE: Management of cardiac arrest. Am Heart J 67:265–277, 1964

35. Johnson J, Kirby CK: Prevention and treatment of cardiac arrest. JAMA 154:291–294, 1954

36. Saltzman GF, Sundstrom KA: The influence of different contrast media for cholegraphy. Acta Radiol [Diag] 54:353–364, 1960

37. Stephenson HE: Yes, Virginia, there is a vasovagal reflex. Chest 64:3–5, 1973

38. Goodman LS, Gilman A: Pharmacological Basis of Therapeutics (ed 4). New York, Macmillan, 1970

39. Lalli AF: Contrast media reactions. Radiology 143:1–12, 1980

40. Johns J: Prevention and treatment of cardiac arrest. JAMA 154:291–294, 1954

41. Phillips JH: Management of cardiac arrest. Am Heart J 67:265, 1964

42. Stanley RJ, Pfister RC: Bradycardia and hypotension following use of intravenous contrast media. Radiology 121:5–7, 1976

43. Andrews EJ Jr: The vagus reaction as a possible cause of severe complications of radiological procedures. Radiology 121:1–7, 1976

44. Witten DM, Hirsch FD, Hartman GW: Acute reactions to urographic contrast medium. AJR 119:832–840, 1973

45. Mann MR: Pharmacology of contrast media. Proc R Soc Med 54:473–476, 1961

46. Rockoff SD: AKERUT contrast media as histamine liberator. Invest Radiol 7:403–406, 1972

47. Lasser EC, Alton JW, Lang JH: An experimental basis for histamine release in contrast material reactions. Radiology 110:49–59, 1974

48. Dean RD, Andrew JH, Read RC: Red cell factor in renal damage from angiographic media. JAMA 187:27–31, 1964

49. Knisley MH, Block EH, et al: Sludged blood. Science 106:431–440, 1947

50. Read RC, Johnson JA, Vick JA, et al: Vascular effects of hypertonic solutions. Circ Res 8:538–548, 1960

51. Almen T, Nordenstam NS: Effects of dyes on microvasculature of the bat wing in vivo. Invest Radiol 4.63 67, 1969

52. O'Connor JF, Sitzman SB, Dealey JB Jr: Vascular injury by topical application of cardiovascular contrast medium. Radiology 89:20, 1967

53. Harrington JH, Wiedman MP: The effect of contrast media on endothelial permeability. Radiology 84:1108–1111, 1965

54. Bjork L: Effect of angiocardiography on erythrocyte aggregation. Acta Radiol [diag] 6:459–464, 1967

55. Meyer MW, Read: Red cell aggregation from concentrated saline and angiographic media. Radiology 82:630–635, 1964

56. Hilal SK (ed): Small Vessel Angiography. St. Louis, C.V. Mosby, 1973

57. Garber GL, Read R: Red cell factor in renal damage from hypertension. Proc Soc Exp Biol Med 107:165–168, 1961

58. Read RC: Cause of death in cardioangiography. J Thorac Cardiovasc Surg 38:685–695, 1959

59. Hilal SK: Hemodynamic changes associated with the intraarterial injection of contrast media. Radiology 86:615–633, 1966

60. Fischer HW: Hemodynamic reactions to angiographic media. Radiology 91:66–73, 1968

61. Foda MJ, Castillo CA, et al: Intravascular pressure response in man to contrast substances used for angiocardiography. Am J Med Sci 250:390–394, 1965

62. Bernstein BF: Respiratory factor in angiographic media toxicity. Radiology 84:670–675, 1965

63. Stein HL, Hilgartner MW: Alteration of coagulation mechanism of blood by contrast media. AJR 104:458–463, 1968

64. Greganti MA, Flowers WM Jr: Acute pulmonary edema after the intravenous administration of contrast media. Radiology 132:583–585, 1979

65. Wood BP, Smith WL: Pulmonary edema in infants following contrast media. Radiology 139:377–380, 1981

66. Dichiro G: Unintentional spinal cord arteriography. Radiology 112:231–233, 1974

67. Kardjiev V, Symeonov A, Chankov I: Etiology, pathogenesis and prevention of spinal cord lesions in selective angiography of the bronchial and intercostal arteries. Radiology 112:81–83, 1974

68. Rhea WG Jr, Dickson J, et al: Multiple injection toxicity of Angioconray. Surgery 55:831–836, 1964

69. Judkins MP, Dotter CT: An uncommon complication of thoracic aortography. Radiology 83:433–435, 1964

70. Berdon WE, Schwartz RH, Becker J, et al: Tamm-Horsfall proteinuria. Radiology 92:714 722, 1969

71. Lang EK, Foreman J, et al: Incidence of contrast media induced acute tubular necrosis. Radiology 138:203–206, 1981

72. Bettman MA, Salzman EW, et al: Reduction of venous thrombosis complicating phlebography. AJR 134:1169–1172, 1980

73. Thomas ML: Gangrene following peripheral phlebography. Br J Radiol 43:528–530, 1970

74. Spigas DG, Thane TT, Capek V: Skin necrosis following extravasation during peripheral phlebography. Radiology 123:605, 1977

75. Gordon IJ: Evaluation of suspected deep venous thrombosis in the arteriosclerotic patient. AJR 131:531–533, 1978

76. Cochran ST, Khodadoust A, Norman A: Cytogenetic effects contrast material. Radiology 136:43–46, 1980

77. Norman A, Adams FH, Riley FR: Cytogenetic effects of contrast media. Radiology 129:199–203, 1978

78. Skovborg F, Nielsen AV, et al: Blood viscosity in diabetic patients. Lancet 1:129–131, 1966

79. Lonni YG, Matsumoto KK, Lecky JW: Post

aortographic cholesterol (atheroma) embolization. Radiology 93:63–65, 1969

80. Jacobsson B, Nillson IM, et al: Catheter material and blood coagulation studies in vitro. Scand J Hematol 6:386–394, 1969

81. Deykin D: Throbogenesis. N Engl J Med 276:622–628, 1967

82. Adams DF, Olin TB, Kosek J: Cotton fiber embolization during angiography. Radiology 84:678–681, 1965

83. Bergeson RT, Rumbaugh CL: Air embolism associated with the use of malfitting plastic connectors in angiography. Radiology 98:689–690, 1971

84. Bove AA, Adams DF, et al: Cavitation at catheter tips. Invest Radiol 3:159–164, 1968

85. Bailey H: Air embolism. J Int Coll Surg 25:675–688, 1956

86. Yune Y, Klatte EC: Fear of angioplasty balloon. AJR 135:395–396, 1980

87. Tegtmeyer CJ, Bezirdjian DR: Removing the stuck, ruptured angioplasty balloon catheter. Radiology 139:231–232, 1981

88. Treatment and reactions to contrast media. Am Coll Radiol 1977

89. Barnhard HJ, Barnhard FM: Emergency treatment of reactions to contrast media. Radiology 91:74–84, 1968

90. Fischer HW, Colgan FJ: Causes of contrast media reactions. Radiology 121:223–227, 1976

91. Robins SL: Pathologic Basis of Disease. Philadelphia, W.B. Saunders, 1974

92. Schwartz CT: Observation of localization of arterial plaques. Circ Res 11:63–73, 1962

93. Crawford T: Some aspect of pathology of atherosclerosis. Proc R Soc Med 53:9–18, 1960

94. Mavor GE: Pattern of occlusion in atheroma of the lower limb arteries. Br J Surg 43:352–364, 1956

95. Gore I, in Anderson WAD (ed): Pathology (ed 5). St. Louis, C.V. Mosby

96. Wagner M, Ricciardi J: A correlative anatomic study of degenerative occlusive disease of the arteries of the lower extremities. Angiology 17:574–582, 1966

97. Lindbon A: Arteriosclerosis of arterial in lower limb. Acta Radiol [Diag] Suppl 80, 1950

98. Haimovici H: Patterns of arteriosclerotic lesions of the lower extremity. Arch Surg 95:918–933, 1967

99. McGarity WC, Logan WD Jr., Cooper WF Jr: Peripheral arterial emboli. Surg Gynecol Obstet 106:399–408, 1958

100. Shumacher HB Jr, Jacobson HS: Arterial embolism. Ann Surg 145:145–152, 1957

101. Wessler G, Schlesinger MJ, et al: Studies in peripheral arterial occlusive disease. Circulation 7:641–655, 1953

102. Warren R, Linton RR, Scannel JD: Arterial embolism. Ann Surg 140:311–318, 1954

103. Lowenberg EL: Changing concepts of the pathology and management of acute arterial occlusion of the lower extremities. South Med J 51:35–42, 1958

104. Baird RJ, Lajos TZ: Emboli to the arm. Ann Surg 160:905–909, 1964

105. Metcalfe WJ: Arterial embolism in the lower limbs. Ann Coll Surg 27:407–426, 1960

106. Flory CM: Arterial occlusions produced by emboli from eroded aortic atheromatous plaques. Am J Pathol 21:549–565, 1945

107. Kazmier JJ, Sheps SG, et al: Liurdo reticularis et digital infarcts. Vasc Dis 3:12–24, 1966

108. Handler FP: Clinical and pathologic significance of atheromatous embolization with emphasis on etiology of renal hypertension. Am J Med 20:366–373, 1956

109. Sieniewicz DJ, Moore S, Moir FE, et al: Atheromatous emboli to the kidneys. Radiology 92:1231–1234, 1969

110. Eliot RS, Kanjuh VL, Edwards JE: Atheromatous embolism. Circulation 30:611–618, 1964

111. Maddison FE, Moore WS: Ulcerated atheroma of the carotid artery. AJR 107:530–534, 1969

112. Sloane L, Allen JH Jr, Collins HA: Radiologic observations in cerebral embolization from left heart myxoma. Radiology 87:262–266, 1966

113. Winkelmann RK, Van Heerden JA, Bernatz PE: Malignant vascular endothelial tumor with distal embolization. Am J Med 51:692–697, 1971

114. Vanway CW III, Lawler MRL: Osteogenic sarcomatous emboli to the femoral arteries. Am J Surg 117:745–747, 1969

115. Christeus N: Embolism to the femoral artery by an echinococcous cyst. Am J Surg 115:673–674, 1968

116. Richey WA: Paradoxical embolism in morbidly obese persons. Radiology 123:43–46, 1977

117. Yatko RD, Trimble C: Arterial bullet embolism. J Trauma 14:200–211, 1974

118. Woodside J, Schwarz H, Bergreen P: Peripheral embolization complicating bilateral renal infarction with Gelfoam. AJR 126:1033–1034, 1976

119. Derrick JR: Clinical and pathological variability in patients with constriction of the superior mesenteric artery. Surgery 52:309–313, 1962

120. Coran AG: Atherosclerosis. N Engl J Med 274:643–648, 1966

121. Leriche R, Moreal A: The syndrome of thrombolic obliteration of the aortic bifurcation. Ann Surg 127:193–206, 1948

122. Starrer F, Sutton D, et al: Aortic occlusion in mitral stenosis. Br Med J 2:644–647, 1960

123. Gilkes R, Dow J: Aortic involvement in Buerger's disease. Br J Radiol 46:110–114, 1973

124. Danto LA, Fry WJ, Kraft RO: Acute aortic thrombosis. Arch Surg 104:569–572, 1972

125. Gross L, Manfredi OL, Fredrick WC: Radiation induced major vessel occlusion. Radiology 93:664–666, 1969

126. Burchmore JW, Goldsmith KLG, et al: Agglutinating sickling arterial thrombosis. Lancet 2:1008–1010, 1962

127. Calem WS, LeVeen HH: Arterial thrombosis complicating inferior vena cava ligation. Surgery 56:612–616, 1962

128. Pader E: Leriche syndrome in a patient with prolonged continued use of ergot derivatives. Vasc Dis 4:380–388, 1967

129. Kramer RA, Hecker SP, Lewis BI: Ergotism report of a case studied arteriographically. Radiology 84:308, 1965

130. Conley JE, Boulanger WJ, Mendeloff GL: Aortic obstruction associated with methysergide maleate therapy for headache. JAMA 198:808–810, 1966

131. Richter AM, Banker VP: Carotid ergotism. Radiology 106:339–340, 1973

132. Kozuka T, Nosaki T, Hara K: Roentgen diagnosis of atypical coarctation of the aorta. Acta Radiol [Diag] 4:497–507, 1966

133. Kozuka T, Nosaki T: Aortic insufficiency as a complication of the aortitis syndrome. Acta Radiol [Diag] 8:49–53, 1969

134. Judge RD, Currier RD, Gracie WA: Takayasu arteritis and the aortic arch syndrome. Am J Med 32:379–392, 1962

135. Thompson JR, Simmons CR, Smith LL: Polymyalgia arteritica with bilateral subclavian artery occlusive disease. Radiology 101:595–596, 1971

136. Rossrussell RW: Giant cell arteritis. Q J Med 28:471–781, 1959

137. Danaras TJ, Wong HO, Thomas MA: Primary arteritis of aorta. Br Heart J 25:153–165, 1963

138. Garland HG: The pathology of aneurysm. J Pathol Bacteriol 35:333–350, 1932

139. Estes JE Jr: Abdominal aortic aneurysm: A study of one hundred and two cases. Circulation 2:258–264, 1950

140. Holman E: Development of arterial aneurysms. Surg Gynecol Obstet 100:599–611, 1955

141. Darling PC: Rupture of arteriosclerotic abdominal aortic aneurysms. Am J Surg 119:397–401, 1970

142. Sommerville RL, Dickson RJ, et al: Bland and infected arteriosclerotic abdominal aortic aneurysms. Medicine 38:207–221, 1959

143. Eastcott HHG (ed): Arterial Surgery. Philadelphia, J.B. Lippincott, 1969

144. Baird RJ, Shivashankar R, Hayward R, et al: Popliteal aneurysms. Surgery 59:911–917, 1966

145. Shucksmith HS: Popliteal aneurysms. Br Med J 1:918–919, 1966

146. Tadavarthy SM, Amplatz K, et al: Syphilitic aneurysm of the innominate artery. Radiology 139:31, 1981

147. Crawford ES, Rambaugh CL, et al: Aneurysm of the abdominal aorta. Surg Clin North Am 46:963–978, 1960

148. Grahal AL, Najaffi J, et al: Ruptured abdominal aortic aneurysm. Arch Surg 97:1024–1031, 1966

149. Jackson RS, Cremin BJ: Angiographic demonstration of gastrointestinal bleeding due to aorto-duodenal fistula. Br J Radiol 49:966–967, 1976

150. Sandler CM, Jackson H, Kaminsky RI: Right perirenal hematoma secondary to leaking abdominal aortic aneurysm. J Comput Assist Tomogr 5:264–266, 1981

151. Lippey EL, Burgh MDC, et al: Concurrent extraperitoneal and intracaval rupture of abdominal aortic aneurysm. Med J Aust 1:517–519, 1978

152. Hershey FB, Spencer AD: Autogenous vein grafts for repair of arterial injuries. Arch Surg 86:836–845, 1963

153. Sawyer JL, Jacobs JK, Sutton JP: Peripheral anastomotic aneurysms. Arch Surg 95:802–808, 1967

154. Wagenvoort CA, Harris LE, et al: Giant cell arteritis and aneurysm in children. Pediatrics 32:861–867, 1963

155. Jofte N: Aneurysm of a persistent primitive sciatic artery. Clin Radiol 15:286–290, 1964

156. Thomas ML, Blakeney CG, Browse NL: Arteriomegaly of persistent sciatic arteries. Radiology 128:55–56, 1978

157. Nicholson RM: Persistent primitive sciatic artery. Radiology 122:687–689, 1977

158. Leading article: Popliteal aneurysms. Br Med J 1:625–626, 1966

159. Giustra PE, Root JA, Mason SE, et al: Popliteal vein thrombosis secondary to popliteal artery aneurysm. AJR 130:25, 1978

160. Wyehulis AR, Spittell JA Jr, Wallace RB:

Popliteal aneurysms. Surgery 68:942–952, 1970

161. Galyis H: Popliteal artery aneurysms. S Afr Med J 48:75–81, 1974

162. Buda JA, Weber CJ, McAllister FF, et al: The results of treatment of popliteal artery aneurysms. J Cardiovasc Surg 15:615–619, 1974

163. Moreno-Cabral R, Kistner RL, Nordyke RA: Importance of calf vein thrombophlebitis. Surgery 80:735–742, 1976

164. Debakey ME, Beall AC Jr, Wukasch DC: Recent developments in vascular surgery. Am J Surg 109:134–140, 1965

165. Smith RF: Arterial trauma. Arch Surg 86:825–835, 1963

166. Smith JW, True aneurysms of traumatic origin in the palm. Am J Surg 104:7–13, 1962

167. Heggelveit HA, Campbell JS, Hooper GD: Innominate artery aneurysms after blunt trauma. Am J Clin Pathol 42:69–74, 1964

168. Abbott WM, Darling RC: Axillary artery aneurysms secondary to crutch trauma. Am J Surg 125:515–520, 1973

169. Swamy S, Segal LI, Mouli SC: Percutaneous angiography. Springfield, Charles C Thomas, 1976

170. Latshaw RF, Weidner WA: Ulnar artery aneurysms. AJR 131:1093–1095, 1978

171. Zak FG, Strauss L, Sophra J: Rupture of diseased large arteries in course of enterobacterial infections. N Engl J Med 158:824–830, 1958

172. Blum L, Keefer EBC: Clinical entity of cryptogenic mycotic aneurysm. JAMA 188:505–558, 1964

173. Debakey ME: Recent developments in vascular surgery. Amer J Surg 109:134–142, 1965

174. Smith RF, Szilagi E, Pffifer JR: Arterial trauma. Arch Surg 86:825–835, 1963

175. Whitaker WG Jr, et al: Acute arterial injuries. Surg Gyn Obst 99:129–134, 1954

176. Wholey M, Bocher J: Angiographic features of aortic and peripheral arterial trauma. Arch Aurg 97:67–74, 1968

177. McKenzie AD, Sinclair AM: Axillary artery occlusion complicating shoulder dislocation. Ann Surg 148:139–141, 1958

178. Bassett FH, Silver D: Arterial injury associated with fractures. Arch Surg 92:13–19, 1966

179. Stone HH, Rutledge BA, Martin JD Jr: Massive crushing pelvic injuries. Amer Surg 34:869–878, 1968

180. Margolies MN: Arteriography in the management of hemorrhage from pelvic fractures. New Engl J Med 287:317–322, 1972

181. Quinby WC Jr: Fractures of pelvis with associated injuries in children. J Ped Surg 1:353–357, 1966

182. Kam J: Vascular injuries in blunt pelvic trauma. Rad Cl N Amer Vol 19, #1:170–176, 1981

183. Miller WC: Massive hemorrhage in fractures of the pelvis: South Med J 56:933–939, 1968

184. Smith K et al: The superior gluteal, an artery at risk. J Trauma 16:273–276, 1976

185. Amato JJ, Rich NM: Temporary cavity effects in blood vessel injury by high velocity missiles. J Cardiovasc Surg 13:147–155, 1972

186. Wilson LB: Dispersion of bullet energy in relation to wound effects. Milit Surg 159:249–256, 1921

187. Gerwig WH, Zimmerman B, Robles NL: Experimental determination of the thermal effects on blood vessels from high velocity missiles. Surgery 59:1065–1068, 1966

188. Peyton RW: Surgical correction of tuberculous pseudoaneurysm of upper abdominal aorta. Ann Surg 162:1069–1074, 1965

189. Holman E in Holman E (Ed): Abnormal Arteriovenous Communications. Springfield, Thomas, 1968

190. Bergan JJ: Basic Surgical Physiology. Chicago, Yearbook Medical Publisher, 1969

191. Holman E: The physiology of an arteriovenous fistula. Amer J Surg 89:1101–1103, 1955

192. Nelson RM, Davis RW: Thoracic outlet compression syndrome. Ann Thoracic Surg 8:437–451, 1969

193. Dick R: Arteriography in neurovascular compression at the thoracic outlet. Amer J Roentgenol 110:141–147, 1970

194. Devillers JC: A brachiocephalic vascular syndrome associated with cervical rib. Brit Med J 2:140–143, 1966

195. Gardner B, Hood RH Jr: Vascular compression at the shoulder girdle. Ann Surgery 153:23–33, 1961

196. Lowe JW, Whelan TJ: Popliteal artery entrapment syndrome. Amer J Surg 109:620–624, 1965

197. Haimovici H, Sprayargren S, Johnson F: Popliteal artery entrapment by fibrous band. Surgery 72:789–792, 1972

198. Gitlitz GF: Anterior tibial compartment syndrome. Vasc Dis 2:122–130, 1965

199. Greenbaum EI: Value of delayed filming in the anterior tibial compartment syndrome secondary to trauma. Radiology 93:373–376, 1969

200. Edwards JE: Congenital heart disease, vol 2. Philadelphia, W.B. Saunders, 1965

201. Colguhen J: Hypoplasia of the abdominal aorta following therapeutic irradiation in infancy. Radiology 86:454–456, 1966

202. Budin JA, Casarella WJ, Harisiadis L: Subclavian artery occlusion following radiotherapy. Radiology 118:169–173, 1976

203. Tracy GD, Ludbrook J, et al: Cystic adventitial disease of the popliteal artery. Vasc Surg 3:10–17, 1969

204. Velasquez G, Zollikoffer CL: Cystic arterial adventitial degeneration. Radiology 134:19–21, 1980

205. Halpern M, Curarino G: Vascular lesions causing hypertension in neurofibromatosis. N Engl J Med 273:248–252, 1965

206. Fleming MP, Miller EW: Renovascular hypertension due to neurofibromatosis. AJR 113:452, 1971

207. Mena E, Bookstein JJ, et al: Neurofibromatosis and renovascular hypertension. AJR 118:39–45, 1973

208. Guilford WB, Pacilio LV: Vascular fracture, new meaning for Monckeberg medial sclerosis. RSNA exhibit, McCormick Place, Chicago, 1981

209. McCormick LJ, Noto TJ Jr, et al: Subadventitial fibroplasia of renal artery, a disease of young women. Am Heart J 73:602–614, 1967

210. Wylie EJ, Brinkley FM, Palubinskas AJ: Extrarenal fibromuscular hyperplasia. Am J Surg 112:149–155, 1966

211. Palma EC: Stenosed arteriopathy of the Hunter canal and loop of the adductor magnus. Am J Surg 83:723–733, 1952

212. McKusick VA, Harris WS, et al: Buerger's disease. JAMA 181:5–12, 1962

213. Lambeth JI, Yong NK: Arteriographic findings in thromboangiitis obliterans. AJR 109:553–562, 1970

214. Randall PA, Blinder RA, et al: Arteria magna revisited. Radiology 132:295–300, 1979

BIBLIOGRAPHY

Abele JE: Balloon catheters and transluminal dilation. AJR 135:901–906, 1980

Adams JT, McEvoy RK, Deweese JA: Primary deep venous thrombosis of the upper extremity. Arch Surg 91:29–42, 1965

Athanasoulis CA: Percutaneous transluminal angioplasty. AJR 135:893–900, 1980

Barth KH, Strandberg JD, White RI Jr: Long term followup of transcatheter embolization with autologous clot oxycel gelfoam. Invest Radiol 12:273–280, 1977

Black AN: Bullet injuries to the arteries. Br Med J 2:872–876, 1964

Block PC, Fallon JJ, Elmer D: Experimental angioplasty. AJR 135:907–912, 1980

Bors E, Conrad CA, Massel TB: Venous occlusion of lower extremities in paraplegic patients. Surg Gyn Obst 99:451–454, 1954

Brockman SK et al: Observation on the pathophysiology and treatment of phlegmesia cerulea dolens. Amer J Surg 109:485–490, 1965

Brodeluis A, Lorenc P, Nylander G: Localization of acute deep venous thrombosis in women taking contraceptives. Radiology 101:297–300, 1971

Castaned-Zuniga WR et al: The mechanism of balloon angioplasty. Radiology 135:565–571, 1980

Cha EM, Khoury G, Waly, FAK: Collateral circulation in superior venacaval obstruction following ventriculo atrial shunt catherization. Radiology 102:605–611, 1972

Chamorro H, Rao G, Wholey M: Superior venacava syndrome: A complication of transvenous pacemaker implantation. Radiology 126:377–378, 1978

Chang J, Katzen BT, Sullivan KP: Transcatheter gelfoam embolization of post traumatic bleeding pseudoaneurysm. AJR 131:645–650, 1978

Cohen LJ et al: Spontaneous aortocaval fistula. Radiology 138:357–359, 1981

Colapinto RF, Harries-Jones E, Johnston KW: Percutaneous transluminal dilatation. Radiology 135:583–587, 1980

Cox JST: Maturation and canalization of thrombi. Surg Gyn Obst 116:593–599, 1963

Cucil CE et al: Venous obstruction of the upper extremity caused by a malformed valve of the subclavian vein. Circulation 27:275–278, 1963

Dible JH: Organization and canalization in arterial thrombosis. J Path Bact 75:1–6, 1958

Dotter CT: Transluminal angioplasty: A long view. Radiology 135:561–564, 1980.

Dotter CT, Judkins MD: Percutaneous transluminal treatment of arteriosclerotic obstruction. Radiology 84:631–643, 1965

Dotter CT, Judkins MD: Transluminal treatment of arteriosclerotic obstruction. Circulation 30:654–670, 1964

Elkin DC: Arteriovenous fistulae. JAMA 134:1524–1529, 1967

Fallon JJ: Pathology of arterial lesions amenable to angioplasty. AJR 135:913–916, 1980

Ferris E: Venography of Inferior Vena Cava and Its Branches. Baltimore, Williams & Wilkins, 1969

Fiddian RV, Byar D, Edwards EA: Factors affecting flow through a stenosed vessel. Arch Surg 88:83–89, 1966

Filshie I, Scott GBD: The organization of experimental venous thrombi. J Path Bact 76:71–77, 1958

Fisher ER: Fibromuscular disease. Arch Int Med 89:343, 1952

Floyd GD, Nelson WP: Developmental interruption of the inferior venacava with azygos and hemiazygos substitution. Radiology 119:55–57, 1976

Gallagher PG, Algird JR: Post radical mastectomy edema of the arm. Angiology 17:377–387, 1966

Gerlock AJ, Muhletaler CA: Venography of peripheral venous injuries. Radiology 133:77–80, 1979

Gibbs NM: Venous thrombosis of the lower extremity with particular reference to bed rest. Br J Surg 45:209–236, 1957

Gralino BJ, Porter JM, Rosch J: Angiography in the diagnosis and therapy of frost bite. Radiology 119:301–305, 1976

Greenfield AJ: Femoral, popliteal tibial arteries: percutaneous transluminal angioplasty. Amer J Roentgenol 135:927–935, 1980

Gruntzig A, Hopff H: Perkutane rekanalisation chronischer arterieller verschlusse mit einem neuen dilatation skatheter. Dtsch Med Wochenschr 99:2502–2505, 1974

Gruntzig A, Kumpe DA: Technique of percutaneous transluminal angioplasty. AJR 132:547–552, 1979

Hansen KF: Idiopathic fibrosis of the mediastinum as a cause of superior venacaval syndrome. Radiology 85:433–438, 1965

Herman RJ et al: Descending venography. Radiology 137:63–69, 1980

Husted JW, Ring EJ, Hirsh LF: Intraarterial nitroprusside treatment for ergotism. AJR 131:1090–1092, 1978

Kaufman SL et al: Transcatheter embolization in the management of congenital arteriovenous malformations. Radiology 137:21–29, 1980

Lagergren C, Lindbom A, Soderberg G: Angiographic demonstration of a tumor thrombus in the popliteal vein. Acta Radiol (Diag) (Stockholm), 52:401–405, 1959

Layne, TA et al: Transcatheter occlusion of the arterial supply to arteriovenous fistulas AJR 131:1027–1030, 1970

Light HG et al: Primary tumors of the venous system. Cancer 13:818–824, 1960

Lindsay SM, Maddison FE, Towne JB: Heparin induced thromboembolism. Radiology 131:771–774, 1979

Lipchik EO, Altman DP: Phlegmesia cerulea dolens. Radiology 133:81–82, 1979

Makin GS: Arterial injuries. Cir Suppl 111:120, 1964

Mann FC, Herrick JF, Essex HE, et al: The effect of blood flow on decreasing the lumen of a blood vessel. Surgery 4:249–256, 1938

Martin EC: AJR 137, 915–918, 1981

Martin EC, Diamond NG, Casarella WJ: Percuta-

neous, transluminal angioplasty in non atherosclerotic disease. Radiology 135:27–32, 1980

Matalon SAT et al: Hemorrhage with pelvic fractures: efficacy of transcatheter embolization. AJR 133:859–864, 1979

May AG et al: Critical arterial stenosis. Surgery 54:259–259, 1963

May AG, Deweese JA, Rob CG: Hemodynamic effects of arterial stenosis. Surgery 53:513–523, 1963

McCormick LJ: Variations in arterial patterns. Surg Gyn Obst 108:149–158, 1959

Negus D et al: Compression and band formation at the mouth of the left common iliac vein. Br J Surg 55:369–374, 1968

O'Dell CW Jr et al: Sodium nitroprusside in the treatment of ergotism. Radiology 124:73–74, 1977

Pillari G et al: Left inferior vena cava. AJR 130:366–367, 1978

Russo PE et al: Changes of the axillary vein after radical mastectomy. South Med J 47:430–436, 1954

Saddekani S, Sniderman KW, Hilton S, Sos TA: Percutaneous transluminal angioplasty of non atherosclerotic lesions. AJR 135:975–982, 1980

Stallworth JM et al: Phlegmesia cerulea dolens, a 10 year review. Ann Surg 161:802–809, 1965

Steinberg I: Thoracic outlet syndromes. N Engl J Med 264:686–692, 1961

Szur L, Bromley LL: Obstruction of the superior venacava in carcinoma of the bronchus. Brit Med J 2:1273–1276, 1956

Tegtmeyer CJ, Buschi A: The angiographic diagnosis of liromyosarcoma of the inferior vena cava. Radiology 122:683–685, 1977

Thomas ML, O'Dwyer JA: A phlebographic study of the incidence and significance of venous thrombosis in the foot. AJR 135:751–752, 1978

Udoff EJ et al: Hemodynamic significance of iliac artery stenosis. Radiology 132:289–293, 1979

Velasquez G et al: Nonsurgical aortoplasty in Leriche syndrome. Radiology 134:359–360, 1980

Virchow, cited in Fontaine R: John Homan's memorial lecture: Remarks concerning venous thrombosis and its sequelae. Surgery 41:6–25, 1957

Walter JF et al: External iliac artery fibrodysplasia. AJR 131:125–133, 1978

Waltman AC: Percutaneous transluminal angioplasty. AJR 135:921–925, 1980.

Wertheimer M, Hughes RK, Castle H: Superior vena cava syndrome. JAMA 224:1172–1173, 1973

Wilder JR, Habermann ET, Nach RL: Subclavian vein obstruction secondary to hypertrophy of the valve. Surgery 55:214–219, 1964

Siddalingappa Srikantaswamy

6

Therapeutic Arteriography: Transluminal Angioplasty

The angiographic catheter that incorporates balloons of variable diameters and lengths[1,2] has become a vital tool in the percutaneous treatment of occluded and stenotic vessels.[3,4]

The underlying principle is overstretching. Intimal cracking and dehiscence of the media allows the encased media to distend, carrying along with it the atheromatous intima. Beyond a certain point, the dilatation will be permanent because of the overstretching of the muscle fibers. The healing process will dress the distended vessel with a scar and line it with a neointima.[5-7]

Balloon angioplasty is an ideal treatment for atherosclerotic stenoses and short occlusions.[8-13] Even aortic thrombosis,[11] fibromuscular dysplasia, and arteritis[14,15] may respond satisfactorily.

A proper clinical evaluation and a knowledge of the patient's subjective symptoms, coupled with noninvasive blood flow studies, are needed to accurately identify the hemodynamic significance of an anatomic lesion. The significance of an anatomic lesion can be further confirmed by measuring pressure gradients.[13] Pressure gradients can be accentuated further by induced vasodilatation. The presence of significant collateral circulation decreases subjective symptoms, but many times it is insufficient during exertion. Arterial stenosis reduces the distal blood flow and pressure only when the critical degree of stenosis is reached. After such a point, even minimal increments of stenosis result in significant drops in distal flow and pressure. The length of stenosis is as important as the percentage of stenosis. The critical percentage of stenosis causing clinical symptoms varies from one circulation to another.[16-19]

Dilatation of occluded segments longer than 8–10 cm, recent thrombosis, heavily calcified vessels, and stenotic small distal vessels may not yield good long-term results. Dilatation of one severe lesion may unmask another significant ipsilateral or contralateral lesion. Such lesions can be dilated when they are clinically obvious. Proximal lesions associated with extremely poor distal circulation may be discouraging, but the results may make a meticulous try at dilatation worth the effort (Figs. 6-1–6-5).

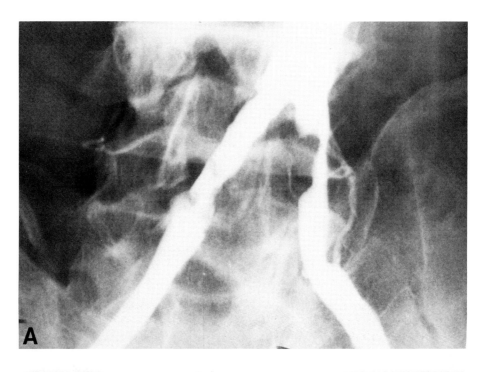

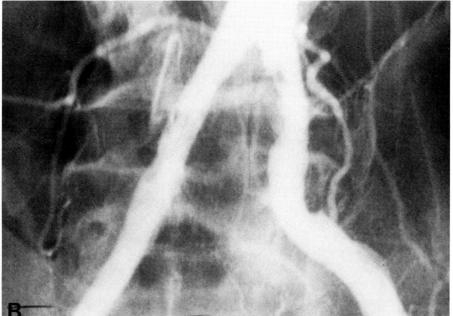

Figure 6-1. Stenotic common iliac artery lesions before (A) and after (B) angioplasty.

144

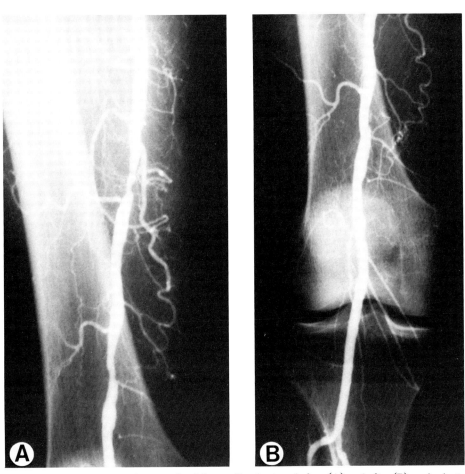

Figure 6-2. Atherosclerotic stenosis of the popliteal artery before (A) and after (B) angioplasty.

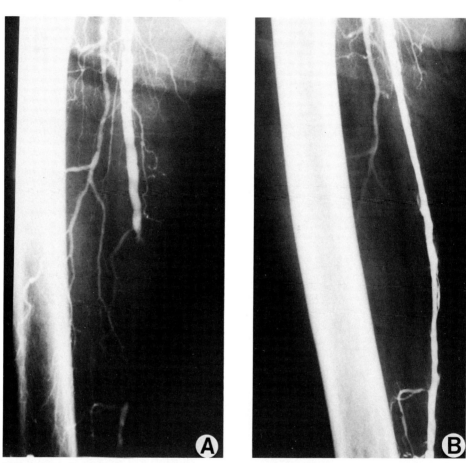

Figure 6-3. Segmental atherosclerotic occlusion of the superficial femoral artery before (A) and after (B) transluminal angioplasty.

146

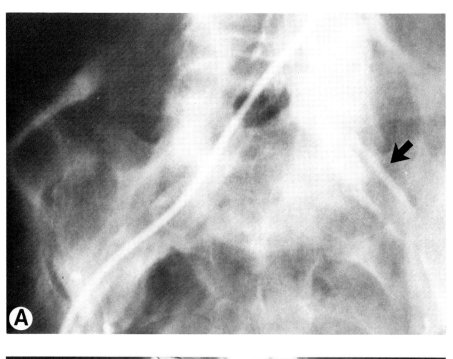

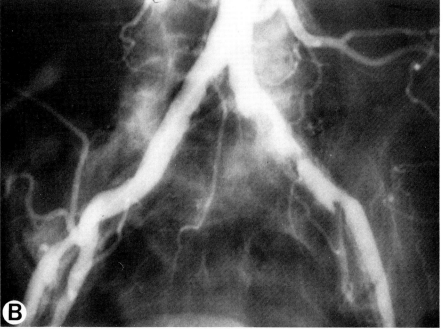

Figure 6-4. (*Continues next page.*)

147

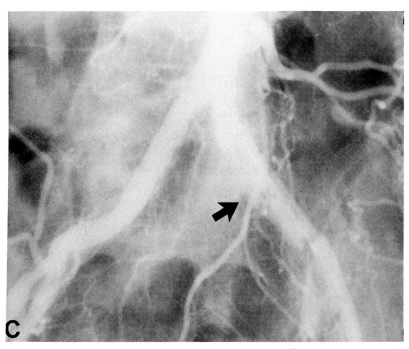

Figure 6-4. (A) A very heavily calcified vessel. Note the unsuccessful angioplasty in B (before) and C (after).

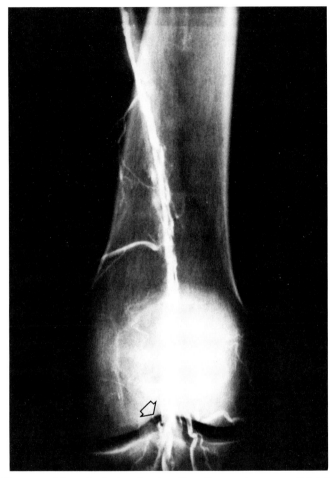

Figure 6-5. Unsuccessful angioplasty of a heavily atheromatous superficial femoral artery. Also note the postangioplasty distal vessel embolization (arrow).

THE BALLOON

The polyethylene catheter balloons with radiopaque markers currently available are very promising. Higher pressures are needed to burst the balloon, since there is no significant stretching, even at the upper limits of operating pressures. Even if it ruptures, the properties of the balloon ensure a longitudinal rather than a circumferential umbrella-like tear. It can be precurved as well as gas-sterilized.[20]

The inflated diameter of the balloon varies from 4 to 6 to 8 mm. Balloon length varies from 3 to 10 cm. Catheter size varies from 5F to 8F. When selecting a balloon, a balloon diameter should be chosen that does not exceed the true normal diameter of the vessel to be dilated. For the smaller blood vessels (e.g., branches of the popliteal artery), a 5F or 6F straight Teflon angiographic catheter will be more than satisfactory. Three to five atmospheres of pressure can be easily generated to expand the balloon with a 2-cc syringe.

COMPLICATIONS

Rupture of the Vessel

Repeated long periods of excessive pressure applied to the balloon will overdistend the vessel and eventually rupture it. The inflated balloon diameter should not exceed the true diameter of the vessel being treated.

Rupture or Detachment of the Balloon

Rupture or detachment of the balloon can be the result of faulty manufacture, repeated inflations and deflations of the same balloon, insertion of a balloon through a subcutaneous scar, or dilating a heavily calcified vessel.

Rupture of the balloon[21,22] can cause severe intimal damage. The balloon may also snag at the puncture site during withdrawal. In the majority of the instances, careful inspection of the balloon before insertion, and replacing the balloon if multiple dilatations are attempted (usually after 4 inflations) will help to avoid balloon rupture.

Recognition of eccentric distension or loss of cylindrical shape suggests impending rupture.

A scarred puncture site should be avoided if possible; if it cannot be avoided, a Desilet Hoffman sheath (Cook, Bloomington, Indiana) should be used for insertion and withdrawal of the balloon catheter.

Opacification of the vessel lodging the balloon while the balloon is being inflated or the return of blood in the catheter while the balloon is being deflated suggests a tear in the balloon. In such instances, the balloon should be immediately deflated and replaced.

Subintimal dissection and occlusion of an adjacent vital collateral vessel may further jeopardize an already diminished circulation. Insignificant distal embolization occasionally can be catastrophic during dilation of an extremely atheromatous vessel.

Guide wire exit through the wall of a vessel in the extremities usually poses no major problems.

TECHNIQUE

A prior knowledge of the patient's clinical and laboratory data (e.g., blood flow studies) is mandatory. This will guide the radiologist in selecting the site (ipsilateral or contralateral) and direction (antegrade or retrograde) for the puncture. This will also enable the radiologist to perform the angioplasty immediately after the angiogram. Antegrade punctures are intended for the ipsilateral femoral and popliteal arteries and their branches. Retrograde punctures are intended for the ipsilateral or contralateral iliac and femoral arteries and the aorta.

After obtaining satisfactory angiograms, the proximal and distal extent of the lesion is located on the skin with radiopaque markers. A 15-mm J wire is inserted through the existing catheter while the catheter tip is maintained 1–2 cm away from the stenotic lesion. By gentle, meticulous manipulation, the true lumen of the stenotic segment is traversed. The guide wire then is advanced further to position the rigid portion of the wire beyond the stenosis. If the segment is occluded, the catheter tip is positioned very close to the occlusion and the occluded segment is probed gently and firmly with the tip of the guide wire. If the 15-mm J wire is unable to traverse the occlusion, a small movable core J wire is used with intermittent stiffening of the tip. Once the guide wire traverses the occlusion, the catheter is advanced beyond the lesion and then is exchanged for the appropriate balloon catheter. The radiopaque markers on the catheter aid in proper positioning of the balloon at the desired level. The balloon is manually inflated under fluoroscopic control using diluted contrast medium. The balloon is inflated for 30 seconds. At this time, 5000 U of heparin is injected through the catheter and the catheter is flushed with normal saline. The balloon is immediately deflated under fluoroscopic control and another arteriogram is obtained. Arteriograms after angioplasty may not always be pleasing because of the intimal splitting and subintimal collection. After proper dilatation, the pulse immediately distal to the puncture site should show definite increases in amplitude on clinical palpation. At a later convenient time, blood flow studies can be done for documentation. Certainly the benefactor (the patient) will eventually compliment or critize the results of the angioplasty. Currently there is no concensus regarding anticoagulant therapy, and it would be difficult to set up a universal regime.[23] Overzealous treatment with heparin causes thromboembolic episodes as a result of thrombocytopenia[24] (see Figs. 6-1–6-5).

Apart from transluminal angioplasty, transcatheter arterial embolization and intraarterial drug infusion have been successfully used in many situations. For intraarterial embolization, various embolic materials have been used.[25] For arteriovenous fistulae, Gelfoam, preoperatively or Gianturco coils for embolization have been used with satisfactory results. Pelvic osseous fractures with associated intractable hemorrhage have been successfully controlled by embolization.[26,27] Intraarterial infusion of nitroprusside for ergotism[28,29] and intraarterial infusion of reserpine in cases of frostbite[30] have been beneficial.

REFERENCES

1. Gruntzig A, Kumpe DA: Technique of percutaneous transluminal angioplasty. AJR 132:547–552, 1979

2. Gruntzig A, Hopff H: Perkutane recanalisation chronischer arterieller verschlusse mit einem neuen dilatations skatheter. Dtsch Med Wochenschr 99:2502–2505, 1974

3. Dotter CT, Judkins MD: Percutaneous transluminal treatment of arteriosclerotic obstruction. Radiology 84:631–643, 1965

4. Dotter CT: Transluminal angioplasty: A long view. Radiology 135:561–564, 1980

5. Castaneda-Zuniga WR, et al: The mechanism of balloon angioplasty. Radiology 135:565–571, 1980

6. Block PC, Fallon JJ, Elmer D: Experimental angioplasty. AJR 135:907–912, 1980

7. Fallon JJ: Pathology of arterial lesions amenable to angioplasty. AJR 135:913–916, 1980

8. Waltman AC: Percutaneous transluminal angioplasty. AJR 135:921–925, 1980

9. Greenfield AJ: Femoral, popliteal, tibial arteries transluminal angioplasty. AJR 135:926–935, 1980

10. Colapinto RF, Harries-Jones E, Johnston KW: Percutaneous transluminal dilatation. Radiology 135:583–587, 1980

11. Velasquez G, et al: Nonsurgical aortoplasty in Leriche syndrome. Radiology 134:359 360, 1980

12. Udoff EJ, et al: Hemodynamic significance of iliac artery stenosis. Radiology 132:289–293, 1979

13. Martin EC, Fankuchen EI: Angioplasty for femoral artery occlusion. AJR 13:915–918, 1981

14. Saddekani S, Sniderman, KW, Hilton S, et al: Percutaneous transluminal angioplasty of nonatherosclerotic lesions. AJR 135:27–32, 1980

15. Martin EC, Diamond NG, Casarella WJ: Percutaneous transluminal angioplasty in non-atherosclerotic disease. Radiology 135:27–32, 1980

16. Mann FC, Herrick JF, Essex HE, et al: The effect of blood flow on decreasing the lumen of a blood vessel. Surgery 4:249–256, 1938

17. May AG, Deweese JA, Rob CG: Hemodynamic effects of arterial stenosis. Surgery 53:513–523, 1963

18. May AG, et al: Critical arterial stenosis. Surgery 54:259–269, 1963

19. Fiddian RV, Byer D, Edwards EA: Factors affecting flow through a stenosed vessel. Arch Surg 88:83–89, 1966

20. Abele JE: Balloon catheters and transluminal dilatation. AJR 135:901–906, 1980

21. Yune Y, Klatte EC: Tear of angioplasty balloon. AJR 135:395–396, 1980

22. Tegtmeyer CJ, Bezerdjian DR: Removing the stuck, ruptured angioplasty balloon catheter. Radiology 139:231–232, 1981

23. Athanasoulis CA: Percutaneous transluminal angioplasty.

24. Fallon JJ: Pathology of arterial lesions amenable to angioplasty. AJR 135:913–916, 1980

25. Barth KH, Strandberg JD, White RI Jr: Long-term follow-up of transcatheter embolization with autologous clot, exycel Gelfoam. Invest Radiol 12:273–280, 1977

26. Matalon S, et al: Hemorrhage with pelvic fractures: Efficacy of transcatheter embolization. AJR 133:859–864, 1979

27. Chang J, Katzen BT, Sullivan KP: Transcatheter Gelfoam embolization of post traumatic bleeding aneurysm. AJR 131:645–650, 1978

28. Husted JW, Ring EJ, Hirsh LF: Intra-arterial nitroprusside treatment for ergotism. AJR 131:1090–1092, 1978

29. Odell CW Jr, et al: Sodium, nitroprusside in the treatment of ergotism. Radiology 124:73–74, 1977

30. Gralino BJ, Porter JM, Rosch J: Angiography in the diagnosis and therapy of frostbite. Radiology 119:301–305, 1976

Gerald D. Pond
Janice R.L. Smith

7
Digital Subtraction Angiography: Technical Aspects

In late 1973 and early 1974, a collaborative effort began between basic scientists and radiologists in an effort to evaluate photoelectronic digital radiography. Since that initial collaboration, a prototype digital video subtraction system has been developed that utilizes state-of-the-art radiographic and computer components.

Photoelectronic radiology includes a wide variety of techniques for image processing covering the entire spectrum of radiologic imaging. Photoelectronic reproductions and manipulation of chest roentgenograms and images of bone structure or vascular anatomy can be performed. Furthermore, because of the active interaction between the cathode-ray tube (CRT) viewing system (television screen) and the digital computer, rapid manipulation of the stored information is possible. By various manipulations and the use of different software programs, objects of interest can be either emphasized or de-emphasized, and the individual preferences of radiologists for image display characteristics can be satisfied.

Digital subtraction angiography (DSA) is only one subtype of the much broader technology of photoelectronic imaging. Digital subtraction angiography applies only to the subspecialty of vascular imaging. The technique primarily is used to evaluate suspected arterial lesions and has the ability to detect suspected lesions of the arteries supplying the head and neck, the renal arteries, the peripheral arteries, and the pulmonary arteries. Digital subtraction angiography has enjoyed rapid technologic advances, not only at the University of Arizona but at many other research institutions in the United States and abroad. The technique is known by many names, including intravenous angiography (IVA), digital video subtraction angiography (DVSA), and photoelectronic intravenous angiography (PIA). It represents the most advanced and most highly developed form of photoelectronic radiology in clinical use today. Although potentially suited to a variety of applications, such as obtaining images of the bones or the lungs and airways, the technique is best suited to evaluation of the human vascular system. Basically, the technique produces excellent images of most arteries without the need for a selective intraarterial injection. The contrast is instead injected intravenously, and the very sensitive detection capability and data manipulation made possible by the computer help to produce diagnostic images. The system is designed to amplify the low contrast levels from iodinated contrast agents up to levels satisfactory for diagnostic interpretation.

Conceptually, the technique is not original or complex. It relies upon the use of subtraction technology and electronically controlled image enhancement to detect low levels of intraarterial contrast. The development of subtraction dates from 1935.[1] The hope was that the amount of contrast needed for an arteriogram could be reduced because of the high toxicity of the original agents employed.[2] By photographically removing extraneous images such as bone and bowel, the low levels of contrast within the vascular system could be more readily identified. The concept of image enhancement also is not entirely new, as anyone familiar with the brightness and contrast controls on a home television set knows. Of course, computer software allows much more sophisticated image manipulations, such as edge enhancement and smoothing. It is apparent that the availability of these high technology, large-memory computers and high-resolution image intensifiers and x-ray tubes were the final ingredients that allowed this technique to develop into its present form.

Even though DSA is a very new technique, diagnostic radiologists and clinicians very quickly accepted it, even though they were initially unaccustomed to vascular images of that type. At our institution, it was only a matter of months before validation studies of the carotid arteries established the accuracy of the intravenous technique. Upon completion of the initial validation studies, vascular surgeons found the intravenous studies to be sufficiently detailed and reliable to serve as the only follow-up angiogram needed postoperatively and later were confident enough to perform surgery based on DSA studies alone. The reason for the rapid acceptance is at least partly due to the proliferation of other imaging technologies, especially those employing a digital computer or a CRT for image viewing. Specifically, recent advances in ultrasound (i.e., real-time) and CT scanning have increased the confidence level of radiologists and clinicians observing representations of human anatomy in these formats. The apprehension about viewing computer processed images, even cross-sections of the body (CT and ultrasound), had disappeared by the time DSA was developed.

Once the reluctance to interpret CRT displays was overcome, the advantages of CRT viewing could be used. Specifically, image manipulations such as filtering, smoothing, subtraction, contrast enhancement, brightness control, magnification, which are accomplished with the speed of the computer allow easy, rapid viewing by the physician. Some clinicians wish to observe manipulation of the data firsthand, although many are satisfied with the image recorded on "hardcopy" (usually 8 × 10-inch film), which is kept in the patient's file.

In selected clinical circumstances, the digital subtraction technique offers many advantages over routine arteriography. Major unique features of DSA, however, are excellent patient acceptance and the fact that it is fast, safe, and much less expensive than a routine study.

To date, DSA is undergoing clinical evaluation at this institution and at several other digital facilities. There are several major areas of interest. These include evaluation of the intracranial and extracranial circulation, primarily in patients suspected of having carotid occlusive disease,[3-8] and diagnosis of suspected renovascular abnormalities, particularly in screening patients for renovascular hypertension, and for preoperative and postoperative evaluation of transplant donors and recipients.[9-14] The technique is also excellent for the evaluation of the thoracic and abdominal aorta[13,15,16] and diagnosis of peripheral vascular occlusive disease.[17,18] The technique has proved valuable for the evaluation of patients who have undergone vascular bypass surgery or angioplasty.[18] Recently, studies indicate that an intravenous injection of contrast can even be substituted for conventional angiograms in cases of suspected pulmonary thromboembolism.[18,19] Many institutions are investigating cardiac applications, including evaluation of contractility, ejection fraction, and chamber and valvular abnormalities.[20-23] Because it is less invasive, potentially one of the most important applications of the digital technique is in the screening of patients for coronary artery disease.[24] Finally, quantitative and qualitative evaluation of blood flow is being examined[25] (Hillman BJ: Personal communication, 1982).

TECHNICAL CONSIDERATIONS AND ADVANTAGES OF DIGITAL SUBTRACTION ANGIOGRAPHY

The digital subtraction facility in use at this institution is an image acquisition system that consists of a high-flux, high-heat-capacity x-ray tube that can deliver multiple short exposures at a rapid rate yet provide adequate x-ray flux for sufficient exposure at the high resolution image intensifier, which is linked by video chain to a digital computer with a very large memory. The computer is interfaced with an analog-to-digital (A/D) convertor. Images obtained by this system are acquired in a fashion similar to that of routine fluoroscopy except for the higher intensity "pulsed" output from the x-ray tube and the higher resolution intensifier, resulting in a signal-to-noise ratio approximately three times greater than that of typical fluoroscopic systems. Images thus obtained are digitized and stored on a disc for "instant" access by both the digital computer for manipulation and the display system for diagnostic viewing. The system block diagram is shown in Figure 7-1.

The system has the capacity to obtain data at rates of up to 30 frames of information per second, a rate equivalent to cinefluoroscopy, and therefore is adequate for cardiac work. Filming rates for some applications, such as peripheral arteriography, only require acquisition rates of one frame per second or less. The television camera used in our system has the ability to generate images that provide in excess of 1500 lines of information, which assures high resolution. Ordinarily, as few as 256 lines of information are sufficient.

The image intensifier is one of the most important elements in the video acquisition chain used for digital subtraction angiography. In addition to high resolution, the field of view is another important consideration. With our original prototype, the image intensifier measured 9 inches in diameter, which allowed only a limited field of view when the size of some areas studied is taken into consideration. Examinations of the lower extremities were not possible using a small intensifier, since the number of runs needed would require a prohibitively large volume of contrast. We have now added a 16-inch, high resolution image intensifier (Thompson, Burbank, CA). Even though the usable field size is actually only 14.5 inches, the intensifier nonetheless expands the field of view significantly. Examinations of the pulmonary circulation, the visceral circulation, and extremity vessels are now feasible. Recently, a prototype

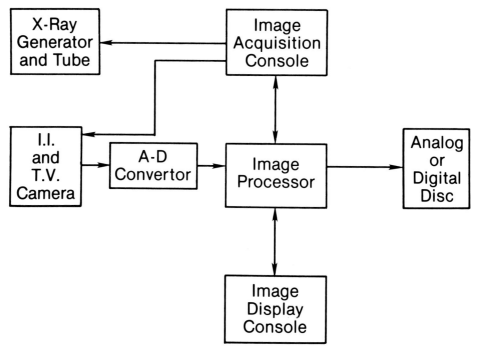

Figure 7-1. Simplified block diagram of a digital subtraction angiographic facility.

22-inch image intensifier has been under development (Siemens, Phoenix, AZ), that will virtually eliminate the problem of a small field of view. Figure 7-2 is a photograph of the current facility at the University of Arizona.

The actual process by which diagnostic images are produced using the digital subtraction technique involves utilization of an image "frame" from the image intensifier before arrival of the contrast bolus into the artery of interest and an image frame obtained when the contrast within that vessel reaches peak concentrations. These two frames are subtracted from one another. The initial frame, before contrast arrival, is known as the "mask" and is subtracted from the image frame at peak concentration, which known as the "raw data" frame. When the two are electronically subtracted, only very faint contrast accumulation can be seen within the arteries. The other structures, such as bone and soft tissues, are subtracted from the area of interest. No subtraction is perfect, however, since motion from respiration, peristalsis, cardiac pulsations, and electronic artifact can all interfere with production of a perfect image. Sometimes these artifacts make the study uninterpretable, and it must be repeated. However, with careful attention to certain technical details and utilization of the means available to minimize problems such as peristalsis (abdominal compression and intravenous glucagon), 85 to 90 percent of studies can be of diagnostic quality.

The computer can be used to salvage some studies using techniques such as "pixel shifts," which can sometimes eliminate an artifact created by 1 or 2 mm of patient motion. Electrocardiographic "gating" during image acquisition and data acquisition at very high frame rates also help overcome some of these difficulties and increase the likelihood of obtaining a close to perfect match between the raw data frame and

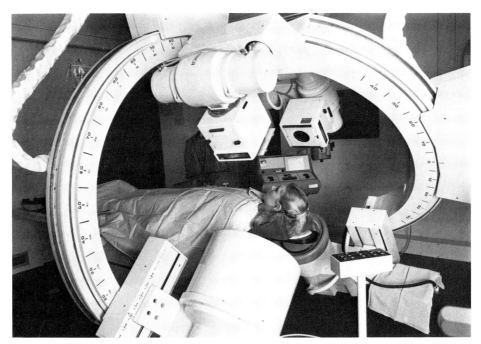

Figure 7-2. A double C-arm facility is shown with the patient in position for a biplane study. The very large 14.5-inch image intensifier is in the foreground. The smaller 9-inch unit is in the background.

the mask frame. The sequence for subtraction and enhancement is shown in Figure 7-3.

During image acquisition, each subsequent image is first preprocessed linearly, by square root, or logarithmically. It is then converted into a digital format and stored (in an effective 256 shades of gray at 2 frames/second). A window location and width within those 256 shades of gray is selected that will correspond to the anatomic point of interest, i.e., the contrast-filled artery. The window width thus is selected so that it corresponds essentially to the contrast level established by the iodine contained in the contrast medium employed, diatrizoate meglumine and diatrizoate sodium (Renografin-76, Squibb, Inc., Princeton, NJ). The window width can either reduce or increase the shades of gray for evaluation. With a narrow window, subtle changes in x-ray attenuation will produce exaggerated changes in the shade as displayed, while an expanded window width will accomplish just the opposite. With a very narrow window, the contrast of the artery is maximized on display. The number of gray levels is increased with wider window settings, but contrast is reduced corresponding to the digital transfer function (gamma) being reduced. The window location is centered generally on the median contrast level, and its width is spread to encompass the range of contrast prevailing in the arterial image. Again the analogy of a television set is appropriate. With each image acquired by the digital unit, a "logo" identifies the various image manipulations that have been performed. This is shown in Figure 7-4.

After the optimal mask and iodinated data frames are selected, subtraction, enhancement, and brightness variation are performed. The various software programs

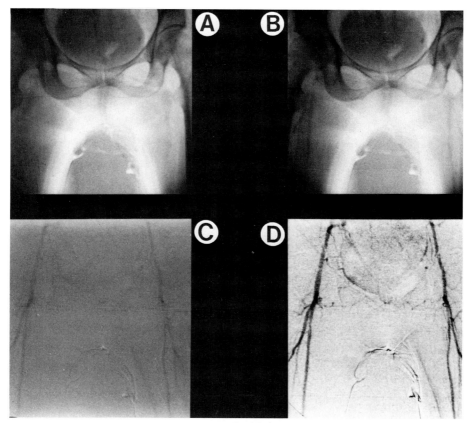

Figure 7-3. (A) A "scout" image centered over the symphysis pubis. A water-filled bag is between the patient's legs to prevent saturation. (B) the "raw data" frame. On careful examination, contrast in the femoral arteries can be seen. (C) Subtraction of the "scout" and "raw data" frames before contrast enhancement better demonstrates the vessels since the bones, contrast-filled bladder, and other structures have been subtracted out. (D) After manipulation of the image, a high-quality arteriographic image is produced.

add to the quality of the image. These include edge enhancement, smoothing functions, magnification, and shifting of mask and data frames relative to one another (pixel shift). The latter is at times most helpful in minimizing (if not eliminating) motion artifacts. Brightness may be varied to visualize more densely opacified structures as well as smaller less conspicuous vessels. Contrast can also be reversed from black on white to white on black. With all of these manipulation techniques available, a particular viewer's image preferences can be satisfied.

In order to obtain a satisfactory digital subtraction angiogram, three conditions must be satisfied. First, there must be no motion during the study, otherwise adequate registration of the mask from raw data images is impossible. Motion can be minimized in a variety of ways depending upon the area being studied: coaching the patient, using abdominal compression, administering drugs such as glucagon to reduce peristalsis, using various immobilization devices, or hyperventilating the patient before breath-holding examinations. Second, a sufficient amount of contrast must be injected

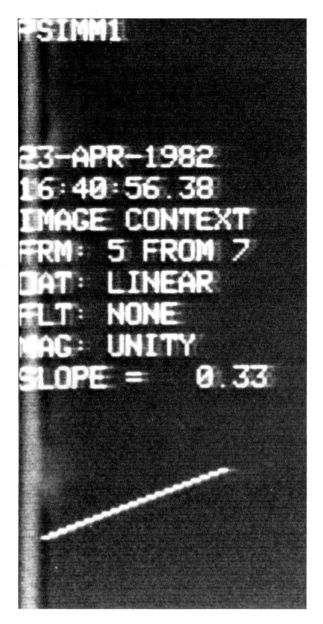

Figure 7-4. A typical "logo" is shown. The identification number and date are at the top. "Image Context" indicates frame (FRM). Frame 5 is the "scout" frame and frame 7 is the "raw data" frame in this example. Data acquisition (DAT) was done linearly in this particular case. Acquisition can also be accomplished utilizing a square root or a logrithmic technique. Filtration (FLT) was not utilized in this patient. Magnification (MAG) was one-to-one. Magnification up to three-to-one is feasible. The slope corresponds to the degree of contrast enhancement.

so that the arterial concentration does not fall below the levels detectable by the digital technique. Hypothetically, this requires a concentration between 0.25 and 0.5 percent, but for practical purposes, concentrations of at least 1 percent are usually needed for quality examinations. Third, photon flux must be sufficient so that the very low contrast levels within the arteries of interest can be discerned from adjacent non-contrast-enhanced anatomy. Generally speaking, all three conditions can be satisfied in about 90 percent of studies.

For intravenous digital subtraction studies, the contrast agent can be delivered by a variety of means. Some institutions prefer utilization of short (4-inch) venous catheters introduced at the antecubital fossa into either the basilic or cephalic vein. The short catheter technique is convenient and very quick, especially at institutions that have a very heavy clinical load, but peripheral injections of this sort carry with them the risk of venous rupture and contrast extravasation into the adjacent soft tissues.[16] With our early cases, we experienced similar problems with the peripheral injection site. At present, our preferred method of contrast administration is via a central venous pigtail catheter placed in the superior or inferior vena cava, although a large number of our patients are now being studied by contrast injections directly into the right atrium. The central technique is somewhat less convenient than a peripheral injection, since a guidewire and catheter must be introduced. We believe, however, that central placement improves the quality of the study, reduces the incidence of some types of technical problems that may arise from a peripheral injection and interfere with diagnosis, and avoids the problem of contrast extravasation. Central contrast extravasation has been known to occur (Tomisch T: Personal communication, 1982), but, in our experience, not when pigtail catheters are used. Of over 1000 patients studied to date, we have as yet not had a serious complication. Virtually all patients experience a sensation of flushing and warmth with each contrast injection, and minor allergic reactions have occurred at an incidence that approximates that expected from routine intravenous urography. Nausea and vomiting occasionally may occur, but this also seems to be of an incidence comparable with that observed with urography. Cardiac monitoring has been performed during both right atrial and superior vena cava injections. In addition, full 12-lead ECGs have been obtained immediately before and immediately after right atrial injections. This was to determine the incidence of cardiac arrhythmias or possible changes in ECG.

The incidence of arrhythmias, usually a single premature atrial contraction (PAC) or premature ventricular contraction (PVC), caused by superior vena cava injections is 13 percent. Right atrial injections have also caused some arrhythmias at a similar incidence (12 percent). The literature reveals that intravenous urography may induce arrhythmias in as many as 33 percent of patients.[26] In one report by Owens and Ennis,[27] 20 percent of the patients had contrast-induced arrhythmias, 12 percent of which were regarded as serious, i.e., ventricular tachycardia. Of the 20 patients who had 12-lead ECGs before and after right atrial contrast injection, no change in the electrocardiogram was noted in any. Based on these data and the subjective impression of improved studies, many more of our intravenous digital subtraction angiograms are being performed utilizing the right atrial injection site. We are now conducting a study comparing the radiodensity over arteries of interest after peripheral or superior vena cava injections with that after right atrial injection. Preliminary data suggests that right atrial injection produces a higher peak concentration and results in denser opacification of the vessel of interest, particularly smaller arteries. The right atrial site appears to be more effective in producing higher contrast concentrations for several reasons. First, the inflowing columns of contrast from the superior and inferior venae cavae tend to confine the contrast bolus within the right atrium, rather than allowing reflux into the innominate, subclavian, and jugular veins, which is commonly observed during peripheral and superior vena cava injections[3] (Seeger JF: Personal communication, 1982). By the same token, the fact that the bolus of contrast occupies much of the volume of the right atrium prevents inflow of nonopacified blood, which would dilute the bolus of contrast. Third, since the atrium is distensible, the contrast bolus causes an end-diastolic volume that is greater than normal, which results in a stronger systole (according to the Frank-Starling effect). This in turn causes increased filling of the right ventricle and by the same mechanism elicits a stronger right ventricular systole.[28] The end result is a nondiluted, more compact bolus of contrast. Contrast volumes injected vary considerably depending on the area of interest, but range from 20 to 50 ml delivered at a rate of 10 to 35 ml sec. Any one of many contrast agents can be used, although we ordinarily employ diatrizoate meglumine (Renografin 76, Squibb, Inc.).

Images are acquired at different rates depending on the area in question. In peripheral vascular studies, rates as slow as 1 frame every other second may be used, whereas cardiac cases require image acquisition rates of up to 30 frames per second. The usual intracranial or visceral study requires from 1 to 6 frames per second depending on the problem for which the patient is being examined.

In addition to digital subtraction angiograms utilizing intravenous injections, digital studies using an arterial injection have also been performed with great success. The major advantage of the digital technique using an intraarterial delivery of contrast is that small vessels, which may not be visualized on a routine arteriogram, can be identified.[17] An intraarterial digital study is routinely able to demonstrate proximally occluded but distally reconstituted arteries. This is particularly important in patients being considered for femorotibial grafts for limb salvage. With the digital technique, reconstituted distal tibial or fibular arteries can be identified and a potential anastomotic site found for the proposed graft.

Intraarterial digital carotid studies have also been performed in patients with intracranial and extracranial neoplastic processes that require embolization. The major advantages of the digital study are that the volume of contrast needed for injection is reduced and that the "instant" subtraction images made possible by the digital technique greatly reduce the time needed to complete the procedure.

With intravenous DSA studies, patients do not require premedication or special preprocedural preparation. Ordinarily, procedures are done on an outpatient basis, resulting in considerable savings since there is no need for extended postprocedural observation (i.e., an overnight stay in the hospital). This saving is in addition to that from the lower cost of the procedure itself, which is approximately one-third that of routine arterial studies. The cost-effectiveness of the digital technique has been verified by several authors.[29-31] The usual digital study is fast, ordinarily requiring only 30 minutes to an hour. Yet another advantage is comfort. Whereas intraarterial injections are often extremely painful,[32] intravenous studies produce only a feeling of flushing and heat. Patient acceptance of the procedure has been excellent because of the comfort, cost, and outpatient status.

Safety is another very important factor in assessing the merits of digital subtraction angiography. Since conventional angiograms require the puncture of an artery, there is a potential for complications such as hematoma, intimal dissection, thrombosis at the puncture site, distal embolization, arterial spasm, and so forth.[33] During cerebral angiograms, there is the additional risk of dislodging an atheromatous plaque or similar complications resulting in stroke. All of these risks of routine angiography are virtually eliminated by the intravenous digital approach.[3-14,34]

The increased safety of intravenous digital subtraction angiography has now made posssible screening evaluations of certain areas of the vascular anatomy by direct visualization.[6,8-11,13,14] This is an important advance. For example, patients with suspected carotid occlusive disease can have a digital study done as a screening test. A routine carotid angiogram could not be justified in that setting in the past because of the risk. Strongly positive indirect studies (Doppler, ophthalmoplethysmography, etc.) or strong clinical evidence had to be present. Since the advent of the noninvasive and cost effective digital technique, patients suspected of transient ischemic attacks (TIAs) can now be examined digitally first. This approach avoids the chances of errors, which are inevitable when the physician is forced to rely on indirect measurements for screening. In patients with suspected renovascular hypertension, screening can be done using DSA. Urography could simultaneously be done by obtaining conventional views after the DSA, just as if a peripheral intravenous injection had been made. Additionally, since a central venous catheter is already in place, the catheter can be advanced and selective renal vein renin samples collected.

One of the greatest potential breakthroughs for digital subtraction angiography is safe screening for coronary artery disease. Again, only indirect indicators such as stress tests are now used for screening to predict coronary disease. Coronary angiography with selective catheterization is too risky to be used as a screening technique. With intravenous injections, screening for suspected coronary stenoses may be possible in the near future.

One important limitation of intravenous DSA needs to be pointed out. Since all of the arteries in the area of interest are simultaneously opacified, overlap of adjacent vessels is unavoidable.[19] Multiple projections can ordinarily overcome this problem, but occasionally a routine arteriogram must be performed because of the failure of the intravenous study. Satisfactory examinations in areas of anatomic interest has been possible in our experience in approximately 85 to 90 percent of patients.[6,9-13]

Several of the major applications of digital subtraction technique are now being examined at this institution. These include evaluation of the intracranial and extracranial carotid circulation, examinations for suspected renovascular abnormalities, study of the aorta and peripheral vessels, imaging of the pulmonary vessels for suspected pulmonary embolism, evaluation of the heart and cardiac chambers, and quantitative assessment of blood flow. In this and the subsequent chapter, the focus will be on the impact of digital angiography on the imaging of the peripheral vascular system.

REFERENCES

1. Ziedses des Plantes BG: Subtraktion: Roentgenographische methode zur separaten abbildung bestimmter teile des objekts. Fortschr Roentgenstr 52:69–79, 1935

2. Fischer HW: Contrast media, in Newton TH, Potts DG (eds): Radiology of the Skull and Brain: Angiography, Book 3. St. Louis, C.V. Mosby, 1974, pp 893–907

3. Chilcote WA, Modic MT, Pavlicek WA, et al: Digital subtraction angiography of the carotid arteries: A comparative study in 100 patients. Radiology 139:287–295, 1981

4. Christenson PC, Ovitt TW, Fisher HD, et al: Intravenous angiography using digital video subtraction: Intravenous cervicocerebrovascular angiography. AJR 135:1145–1152, 1980

5. De Lahitte MD, Marc-Vergres JP, Roscol A, et al: Intravenous angiography of the extracranial cerebral arteries. Radiology 137:705–711, 1980

6. Seeger JF, Weinstein PR, Carmody RF, et al: Digital video subtraction angiography of the cervical and cerebral vasculature. J Neurosurg 56:173–179, 1982

7. Modic MT, Weinstein MA, Chilcote WA, et al: Digital subtraction angiography of the intracranial vascular system: Comparative study in 55 patients. Am J Neuroradiol 2:527–534, 1981

8. Buonocore E, Meaney TF, Borkowski GP, et al: Digital subtraction angiography of the abdominal aorta and renal arteries. Radiology 139:281–286, 1981

9. Hillman BJ, Ovitt TW, Capp MP, et al: The potential impact of digital video subtraction angiography on screening for renovascular hypertension. Radiology 142:577–579, 1982

10. Hillman BJ, Ovitt TW, Nudelman S, et al: Digital video subtraction angiography of renal vascular abnormalities. Radiology 139:277–280, 1981

11. Hillman BJ, Smith JRL, Pond GD, et al: Current Radiology: Photoelectronic Radiology. Baltimore, Williams & Wilkins, 1982

12. Osborne RW Jr, Goldstone J, Hillman BJ, et al: Digital video subtraction angiography: Screening technique for renovascular hypertension. Surgery (in press, 1982)

13. Pond GD, Smith JRL, Hillman BJ, et al: Current clinical applications of digital subtraction angiography. Appl Radiol 10:71–79, 1981

14. Smith CW, Winfield AC, Price RR, et al: Evaluation of digital venous angiography for the diagnosis of renovascular hypertension. Radiology 144:51–54, 1982

15. Sahn DJ, Pond GD, Allen HD, et al: Evaluation of aortic arch abnormalities and pulmonary artery anatomy by intravenous digital subtraction angiography and 2D echo. Presented at the 55th Annual Meeting of the American Heart Association, Dallas, Texas, November 15, 1982

16. Meaney TF, Weinstein MA, Buonocore E, et al: Digital subtraction angiography of the human cardiovascular system. AJR 135:1153–1160, 1980

17. Crummy AB, Strother CM, Liebermann RP, et al: Digital video subtraction angiography for evaluation of peripheral vascular disease. Radiology 141:33–37, 1981

18. Pond GD, Osborne RW, Capp MP, et al: Digital subtraction angiography of peripheral vascular bypass procedures. AJR 138:279–282, 1982

19. Pond GD, Cook GC, Woolfenden JM, et al: Pulmonary thromboembolism: Evaluation by digital intravenous angiography. Proceedings of the Society of Photo-optical Instrumentation Engineers 314:256–262, 1981

20. Kruger RA, Anderson RE, Koehler R, et al: A method for the noninvasive evaluation of cardiovascular dynamics using a digital radiographic device. Radiology 139:301–305, 1981

21. Erikson U, Helmius G, Hennig K, et al: Determination of myocardial blood flow by videodensitometry. Fortschr Roentgenstr 135:404–406, 1981

22. Kruger RA, Mistretta CA, Houk TL, et al: Computerized fluoroscopy techniques for intravenous study of cardiac chamber dynamics. Invest Radiol 14:279–287, 1979

23. Carey PH, Slutsky RA, Ashburn WL, et al: Validation of cardiac output estimates by digital video subtraction angiography in dogs. Radiology 143:623–626, 1982

24. Patton DD, Pond GD: Digital subtraction angiography: Impact on nuclear medicine, in Harbert J, de Roche A (eds): Textbook of Nuclear Medicine: Clinical Applications. Philadelphia, Lea & Febiger, 1982

25. Buersch JH, Hahne HJ, Brennecke R, et al: Assessment of arterial blood flow measurements by digital angiography. Radiology 141:39–47, 1981

26. Berg GR, Hutter AM Jr, Pfister RC: Electrocardiographic abnormalities associated with intravenous urography. N Engl J Med 289:87–88, 1973

27. Owens A, Ennis M: Arrythmias occurring during intravenous urography. Clin Radiol 31:291–295, 1980

28. Goldman S, Olajos M, Morkin E: Effects of verapamil on positive inotropic stimulation in the left atrium and ventricle of conscious dogs. J Pharm Exp Ther (in press)

29. Freedman GS: Economic analysis of outpatient digital angiography. Appl Radiol 11:29–38, 1982

30. Dwyer SJ III, Templeton AW, Martin NL, et al: The cost of managing digital diagnosis images. Radiology 144:313–318, 1982

31. Detmer DE, Fryback DG, Strother CM: Digital subtraction arteriography cost-effectiveness, in Mistretta CA, Crummy AB, Strothers CM, et al (eds): Digital Subtraction Arteriography. Chicago, Year Book, 1982

32. Guthaner DF, Silverman JF, Mayden WG, et al: Intra-arterial analgesia in peripheral arteriography. AJR 128:737–739, 1977

33. Sigstedt B, Lunderquist A: Complications of angiographic examinations. AJR 130:455–460, 1978

34. Weinstein MA, Modic MT, Buonocore E, et al: Digital subtraction angiography: Experience at the Cleveland Clinic Foundation. Appl Radiol 10:53–66, 1981

Gerald D. Pond
Janice R.L. Smith

8
Digital Subtraction Angiography of the Extremities

Arteriograms of the extremities are perhaps one of the most commonly requested angiographic procedures. The most common indications are lower extremity ischemia, especially debilitating claudication; non-healing ulcers; or impending loss of a digit or limb. Although the most common etiologic cause for the ischemia is atherosclerosis, many patients are studied for other vascular disorders that may have ischemic symptomatology such as Raynaud's phenomenon, Mönckeberg's medial calcific sclerosis, Buerger's disease, and peripheral emboli. In addition to evaluating patients with ischemia, patients with hemodialysis shunts, suspected arteriovenous malformations or fistulae, and abdominal aortic or peripheral aneurysms are also studied.

An extremity arteriogram serves several basic functions. It may help to determine the etiology of the symptoms. It may determine whether the vascular abnormality is treatable, and also provides an anatomic "roadmap." It thus may establish the cause, the extent and location, the feasibility of treatment of the disease process, and the type of treatment applicable, be it angioplasty, embolotherapy, surgery, or some other alternative.

Routine arteriography requires that access to the vascular system be made by arterial puncture, usually the femoral artery. Occasionally, less preferable approaches are necessary, such as axillary angiography or translumbar aortography. The risks of routine arteriography are well known.[1,2] Complications at the puncture site, such as hematoma, thrombosis, distal embolization as a result of dislodgement of a plaque, arterial spasm, etc., require careful observation after the procedure. Patients ordinarily require overnight hospitalization. Since arteriograms are performed by highly trained subspecialists and requires a great deal of technical support as well as sophisticated equipment, these procedures are expensive.[3,4] Added to that expense is the need for hospitalization for a study to be completed.

Most patients regard arteriography as an unpleasant experience. Some patients may be reluctant or even refuse to undergo a second study. This is probably because of the pain of extremity arteriography, which some patients describe as excruciating.[5] Even intraarterial analgesics such as lidocaine do not completely overcome this problem during routine arteriography.[6]

In selected patients, the basic objectives of routine extremity arteriography can be accomplished using the alternative digital intravenous method. The technique produces images of the peripheral arteries that are very often comparable in quality to those obtained by conventional techniques.[7] In addition, the procedure is safer, requiring no arterial puncture, since contrast is administered into a vein.[7] Studies can be performed on an outpatient basis, thereby reducing the cost to approximately one-third that of a conventional examination.[8] Because of safety, cost, and less discomfort, patient acceptance is excellent.

The amount of technical expertise required to perform a satisfactory intravenous digital subtraction angiogram is less than that required for conventional angiography. This may ultimately permit angiography to be performed on a limited basis in smaller hospitals and in some outpatient facilities by radiologists without the sophisticated training now needed to perform conventional angiograms.

In addition to the digital subtraction angiograms performed after intravenous injections, digital subtraction angiography performed using intraarterial injection of contrast offers advantages over conventional techniques. Very small vessels, which cannot be seen on conventional angiograms, can often be seen using the digital approach.[7,10] Intraarterial digital studies require less contrast, yet still provide good visualization of vessels. This reduces the degree of discomfort experienced by the patient.

METHOD

The technique for intravenous digital examinations of the extremities is the same as that used for other areas of the vascular anatomy. A vein in the antecubital fossa is selected, and after venipuncture, a guidewire is introduced. This is followed by placement of a pigtail catheter into a central venous location, usually the superior vena cava or right atrium. Contrast volumes vary according to such factors as cardiac output and the size of the patient, but average approximately 40 ml delivered over 2 seconds. Film rates vary between 2 frames per second for examinations of the distal abdominal aorta and 1 frame every other second for examinations of the smaller distal vessels of the upper or lower extremity.

The images are usually obtained using a 14.5-inch image intensifier, which allows the largest possible field of view. For comprehensive "runoff" studies, this reduces the total number of injections required and minimizes contrast volume. For most patients, when evaluation from the renal arteries to the popliteal "trifurcation" is desired, four views are necessary. For examinations of the hand or foot, such as in Raynaud's phenomenon, a smaller intensifier is adequate.

Three conditions must be satisfied in order to obtain a satisfactory digital examination. First, the concentration of contrast medium must be sufficient to be detectable by the digital technique. We consistently have been able to visualize even the most distal of the extremity vessels with relatively small amounts of contrast—never more than 40 ml. We are currently experimenting with further diminution in contrast volumes. Second, photon flux must be sufficient so that the very low contrast levels can be demonstrated and discerned from adjacent nonenhanced anatomy. In all but the most obese of patients, we are able to satisfy this condition. Third, motion must be minimized. Motion is generally not a problem when evaluating the extremities, since immobilizing the arms or legs is not difficult. Patients who are completely uncooperative, however, may be able to move the lower extremity so much that accurate "registration" of the scout and data frames is not adequate for subtraction. Even cooperative patients may move slightly. This slight motion produces a linear artifact that corresponds to the margin of the bone cortex. These artifacts can make interpretation difficult, since the high-density artifacts are usually oriented in the same direction as the vessels being studied. The utilization of "pixel shift" often can overcome the problem, and the study can be salvaged.

Another problem related to artifact is encountered when comprehensive evaluation of the abdominal aorta and peripheral runoff is needed. This artifact is peristaltic motion, which sometimes is not overcome even with intravenous administration of glucagon and compression of the abdomen. Satisfactory images sometimes simply cannot be obtained. In our experience, diagnostic abdominal images are nonetheless produced in over 85 percent of studies.

For intraarterial digital subtraction angiography, an Amplatz sheath (Cook, Bloomington, IN) is introduced. If desired, a single-wall puncture can be made. Contrast is then injected through the sheath, and images are obtained over the area of interest. Filming rates vary between 2 per second and 1 every other second. For examinations of the hand, we use a low brachial artery injection. For examinations of the lower extremity, the femoral artery is used.

The views obtained vary greatly and depend on the disease condition for which the patient is being studied. For evaluation of peripheral runoff, anteroposterior (AP) projections are used, and steep oblique views are added when the profunda femoris arteries are not well seen on the AP views. For evaluation of the smallest distal vessels, such as digital arteries, anteroposterior or lateral views of the hand or foot may be needed.

RESULTS

When all the types of extremity studies that have been performed are considered, diagnostic examinations have been possible in over 90 percent. The most common causes of an unsuccessful examination have been failure of the patient to fully cooperate and peristaltic motion that could not be adequately suppressed with glucagon and compression. We have learned that patients who cannot or will not cooperate for DSA should be examined by conventional techniques. The chances of obtaining a successful examination on unwilling patients are extremely remote. Very active peristalsis has interfered predominantly in evaluation of the distal aorta and iliac vessels. Twenty-two of the first 25 digital aortofemoral runoff studies have been successful (88 percent). The other three were compromised by peristalsis.

Extremity studies have been successful in a remarkable percentage of cases. In our first 38 studies in patients who had undergone peripheral bypass surgery, every examination was diagnostic. The digital studies were confirmed by routine angiography, intraoperative arteriography, or surgical findings.[7] Even complex grafts are well demonstrated consistently. The intraarterial studies have also been of reliable

diagnostic quality, and although the absolute number of examinations we have performed to date is relatively small, this impression is in keeping with the experience
of others.[9]

CLINICAL EXAMPLES OF DIGITAL SUBTRACTION
ANGIOGRAPHY OF THE EXTREMITIES

Abdominal Aortography with Lower Extremity
Arteriography

When the only high-resolution image intensifier available in our system had a
maximal viewing area of 9 inches, comprehensive examination of the abdominal aorta
and peripheral vessels was not feasible. The field size covered on a single injection
was simply not large enough. Even if a hypothetical patient weighing 50 k and standing
150 cm high is considered, approximately 60 cm of body length would have to be
examined for an adequate study. A minimum of three separate injections would be
required to study just one side. The width of the intensifier also is 9 inches (approximately 23 cm). A bilateral study could not be done with such a small intensifier face,
and a complete examination would therefore require a minimum of five injections.
Since the average contrast volume used is 40 ml, the total needed to complete the
study would be 200 ml. In this hypothetical patient, 4 ml of contrast per kilogram
of body weight would have been given, which is a very large volume and much more
than that would be given during a conventional study. If additional views were
necessary, toxic levels of contrast could be reached.

Because of the limitation imposed by the small intensifier, initial studies of the
peripheral vessels were of limited anatomic areas, such as the region of known lesions,
i.e., an abdominal aortic aneurysm (Fig. 8-1) or at a suspected stenosis or occlusion.

With the new, larger intensifier, the field-of-view problem appears to be largely
resolved. For most patients, three to four imaging runs visualize the abdominal aorta
and the lower extremity arterial supply. The width intensifier is also adequate to study
both legs simultaneously. The contrast volume required is therefore acceptable, usually
between 120 and 160 ml. Figures 8-2, 8-3, and 8-4 show composites of runoff studies
obtained with the larger intensifier.

Although the early experience with intravenous DSA of the aorta and peripheral
vessels has been encouraging, it is not yet possible to suggest that DSA will eliminate
the need for conventional angiography preoperatively. Additional investigation is
underway to determine the overall accuracy in large numbers of patients. There are
some situations, however, in which the intravenous digital study is the first choice.
Some patients who have undergone many vascular bypass procedures have little or
no remaining access to the arterial system. Translumbar aortography was the only
option in some of these patients until the advent of the digital technique. When a
satisfactory examination cannot be obtained for any anatomic or technical reason,
DSA is an appealing alternative.

There are limitations in DSA studies of the abdominal aorta. Already mentioned
is peristaltic artifact (Figs. 8-3, 8-5). Another limitation is contrast volume, which
usually exceeds that which would be administered during conventional studies. This
limitation may be outweighed by the advantages of not using an arterial access site

for the examination. In patients with very large abdominal aortic aneurysms, the contrast volumes required for adequate visualization are prohibitively large in many cases. This is principally because of the hemodilution occurring within the aneurysm, which acts something like a reservoir. It is best to study these patients with conventional technique.

The diagnostic quality of the digital subtraction angiograms, be they limited-field studies or full-field studies, often produce angiographic images of near comparable quality to conventional images (Figs. 8-6, 8-7).

Evaluation of Patients After Bypass Surgery

One of the largest groups of patients in whom digital subtraction angiograms have been performed for peripheral vessels are those who have undergone bypass surgery. When symptomatic improvement after surgery is less than anticipated, the question of graft thrombosis or other complications may arise. Intravenous DSA offers significant advantages in this situation. The patient is spared a repeat conventional angiogram, grafts need not be punctured, and recent operative sites can be avoided. Similarly, if patients have had a functioning bypass graft and later experience a change in symptomatology, the graft can be evaluated using the digital approach. In our original series of 30 examinations of bypass grafts, in which patients had confirmatory conventional or intraoperative angiography or the findings were confirmed by subsequent surgery, DSA was correct in every case.[7] Figures 8-8 and 8-9 are examples of patent bypass grafts. Figure 8-10 is an example of a thrombosed axillofemoral graft and also shows some of the image manipulations possible using the DSA system. Routinely, grafts are examined at both their proximal and distal anastomoses. Although most grafts will occlude completely from their origin to the distal anastomosis, some thrombi may not as yet be fully formed. One end of a graft may still partially fill. Failure to demonstrate patency at both ends of the graft confirms occlusion.

Intravenous DSA for Suspected Embolism

Defining the location and extent of a suspected peripheral embolus is extremely important whenever thrombolytic therapy or surgical intervention is required. Again, DSA eliminates the need to perform an arterial puncture and to place a catheter, thus avoiding the risk of dislodging embolic material. Figures 8-11 and 8-12 are examples of emboli detected by intravenous DSA.

Detection of Peripheral Aneurysms, Arteriovenous Malformations and Arteriovenous Fistulae

Yet another application of DSA we find to be of value is in defining suspected aneurysms, arteriovenous fistulae, and arteriovenous malformations of peripheral vessels. Figure 8-13A demonstrates a traumatic pseudoaneurysm produced after arterial puncture for cardiac catheterization. Arteriovenous malformations and fistulae are also identifiable using the digital subtraction technique, especially when the flow rates through these lesions is high. Predominately venous vascular malformations are less well visualized because of slow flow and hemodilution.

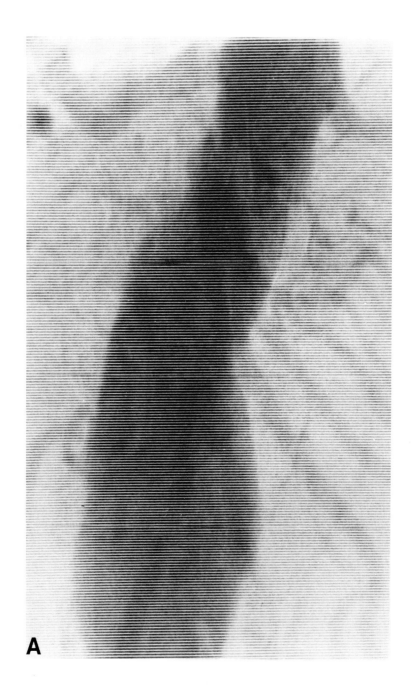

A

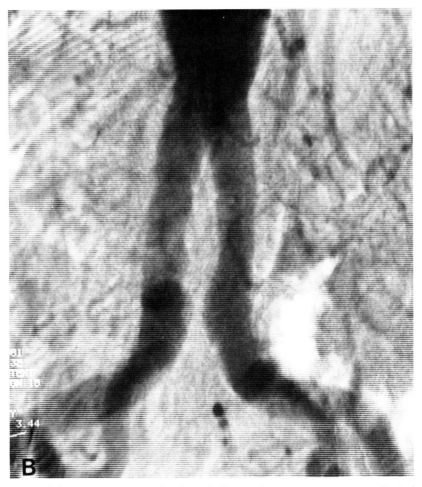

Figure 8-1. (A) A digital study of the abdominal aorta demonstrates patent renal arteries and an abdominal aortic aneurysm. Note the very limited field of view in this study, which was done on a 9-inch intensifier. Only regional studies are possible with small intensifiers. (B) The distal end of the aorta is seen. The aneurysm does not involve the iliac arteries.

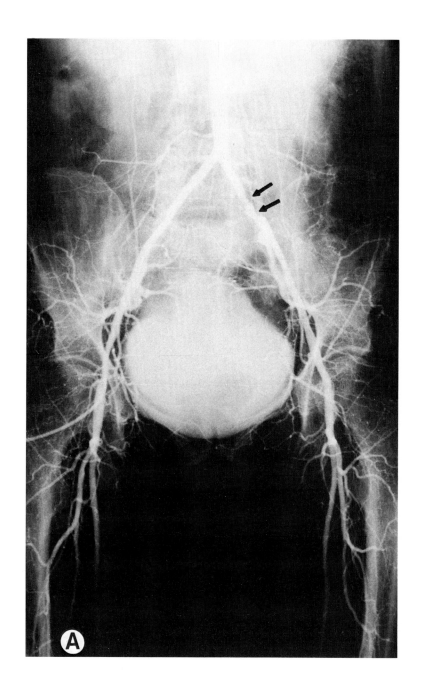

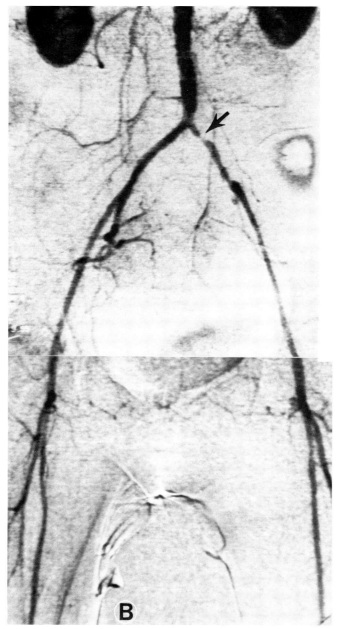

Figure 8-2. (A) A conventional arteriogram shows two stenoses of the left internal iliac (arrows). (B) A composite of two digital intravenous studies of the same patient done 2 years later demonstrates the extended field of view of the 14.5-inch intensifier. The two stenoses of the left common iliac artery are again well seen. However, a new and more proximal lesion is now present (arrow).

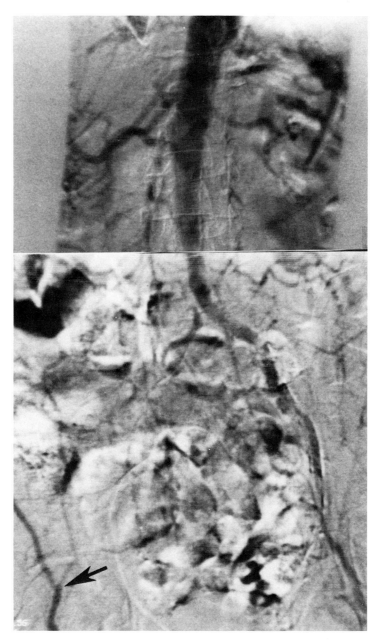

Figure 8-3. A composite of two digital intravenous studies of the aorta and pelvic vessels shows both renal arteries and the complete occlusion of the right common iliac. The site of reconstitution is well demonstrated (arrow). Note the peristaltic artifact, which compromises the visualization of the left iliac arteries.

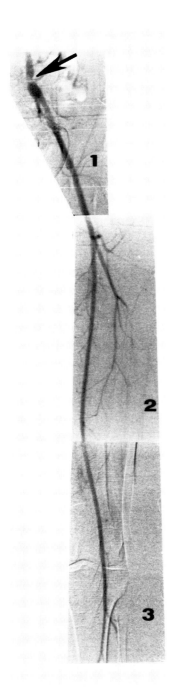

Figure 8-4. A composite of three digital intravenous studies shows a tight stenosis of the common iliac artery (arrow). The remainder of the runoff down to the level of the popliteal "trifurcation" is normal.

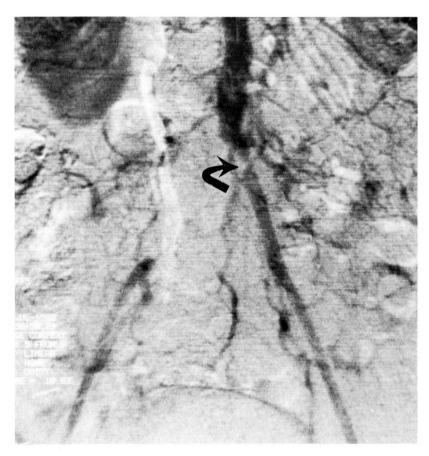

Figure 8-5. Another study of the pelvic vessels demonstrates complete occlusion of the right common iliac artery with distal reconstitution. There is also a high grade stenosis of the proximal left common iliac artery (arrow). The artifact in this case is caused by peristalsis but is minimal.

176

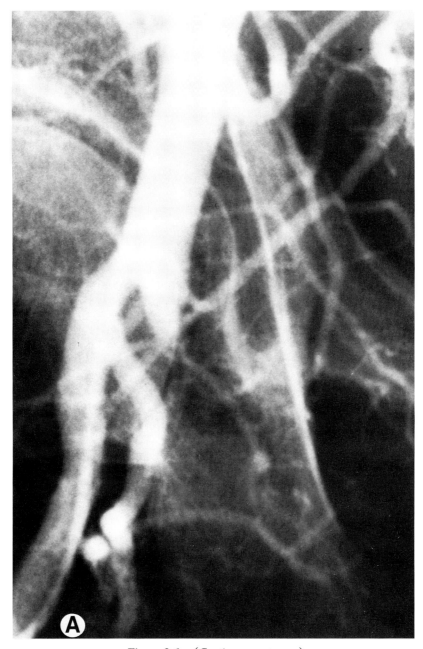

Figure 8-6. (*Continues next page.*)

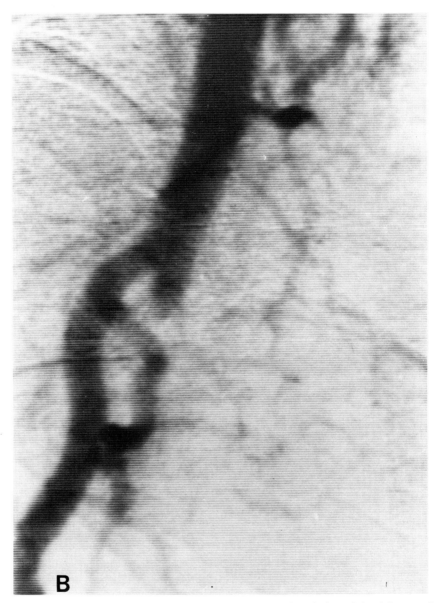

B

Figure 8-6. (A) A conventional angiogram demonstrates total occlusion of the right superficial femoral artery. (B) The intravenous digital subtraction angiogram of the same anatomic location is of near comparable quality to the conventional study.

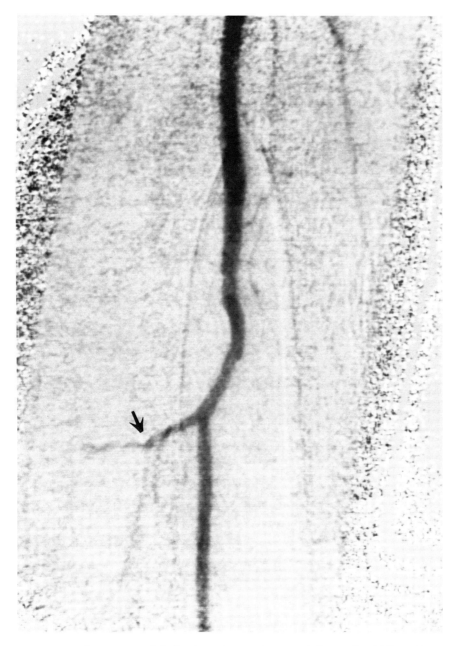

Figure 8-7. An intravenous digital subtraction angiogram of the popliteal bifurcation demonstrates complete occlusion of the anterior tibial artery (arrow).

179

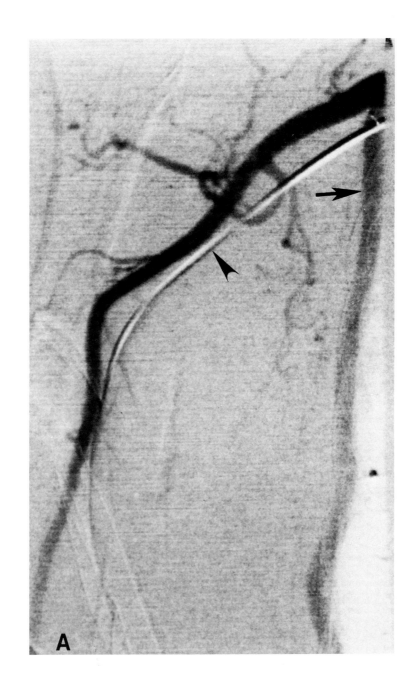

A

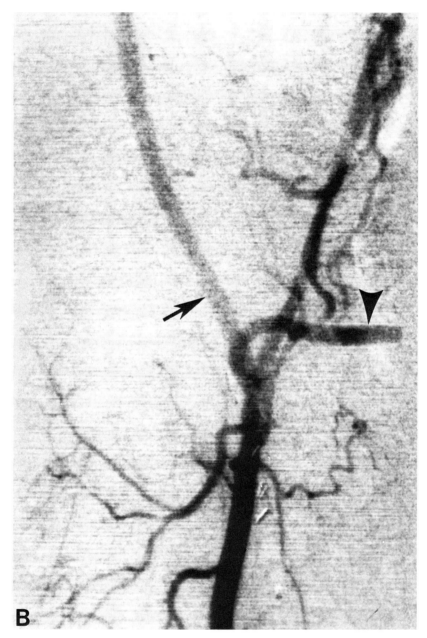

B

Figure 8-8. (A) An intravenous digital subtraction angiogram including the origin of an axillofemoral graft from the right axillary artery is shown (arrow). Note the image of the catheter, passing through the basilic and axillary veins (arrowhead). (B) The distal anastomosis of the patient's axillofemoral graft is demonstrated (arrow). The proximal limb of a femoro-femoral graft (arrowhead) is also clearly demonstrated. The native external iliac artery filled in a retrograde direction.

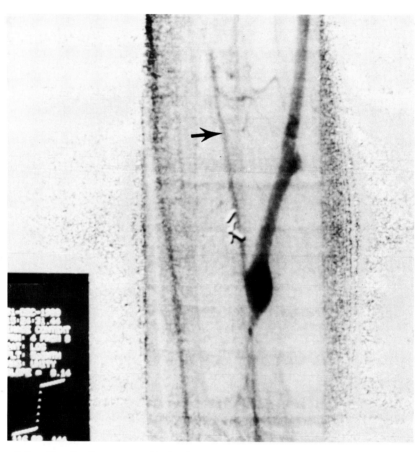

Figure 8-9. The distal anastomosis of a femoroposterior tibial graft is clearly demonstrated. There is also retrograde filling of the native posterior tibial artery (arrow).

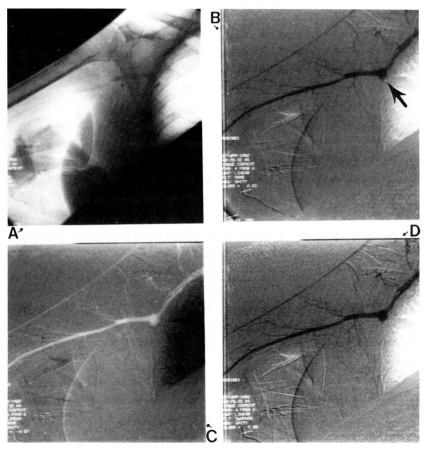

Figure 8-10. An example of typical "hard copy" is shown. The DSA images are of the right axilla and include scout (A), black-on-white (B), white-on-black (C), and "smoothed" black-on-white versions (D). The site of a now-thrombosed axillofemoral graft is shown (arrow). The curvilinear artifact seen on the subtracted images is produced by slight motion of the patient's breast, which can also be seen in the scout data frame.

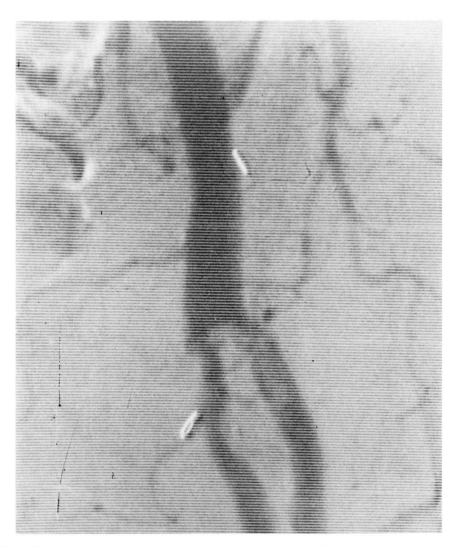

Figure 8-11. An intravenous digital subtraction angiogram of the left common femoral artery demonstrates a filling defect. The patient was in atrial fibrillation and developed acute left lower extremity ischemia consistent with embolic occlusion.

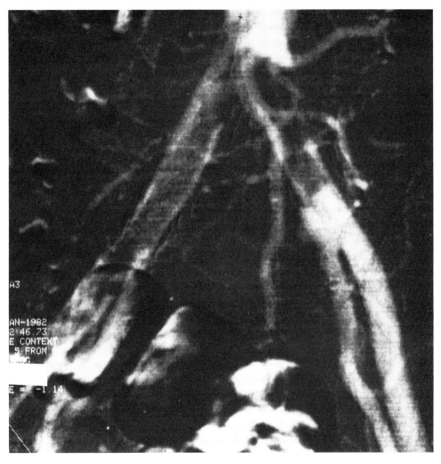

Figure 8-12. A saddle embolus of the distal aorta and proximal iliac vessels is demonstrated on an intravenous digital subtraction study.

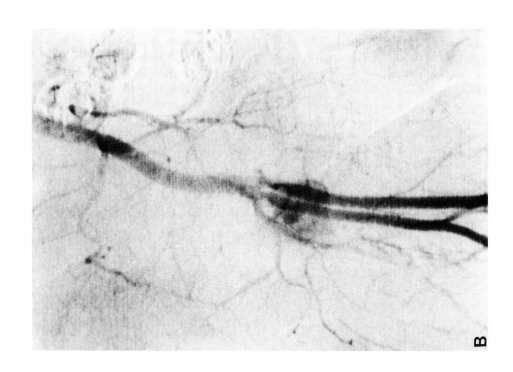

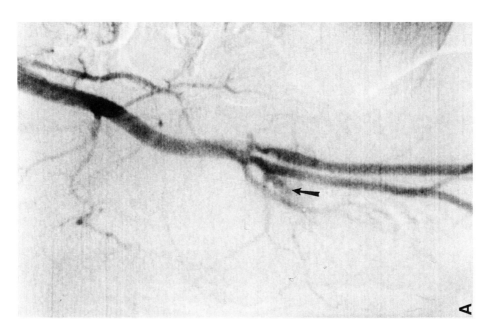

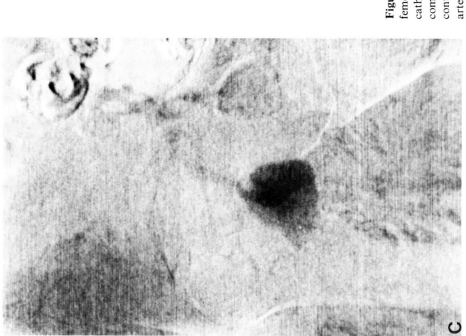

C

Figure 8-13. (A) An intravenous digital subtraction angiogram of the right common femoral artery in a patient who had developed a pulsatile groin mass after cardiac catheterization. Note the small amount of contrast extravasation from the region of the common femoral bifurcation (arrow). (B) An image made somewhat later shows more contrast extravasation. (C) A large accumulation of contrast is now apparent after arterial washout. The diagnosis of iatrogenic pseudoaneurysm was made.

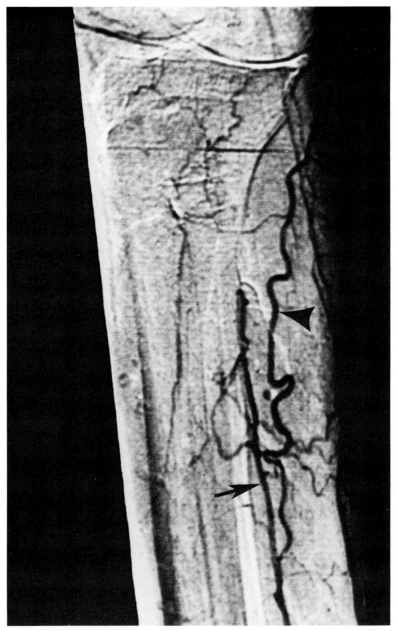

Figure 8-14. A conventional angiogram had failed to demonstrate any of this patient's "trifurcation" vessels. The intraarterial digital subtraction angiogram shows a patent posterior tibial artery (arrow) that was reconstituted by a tortuous collateral (arrowhead).

Demonstration of Small Distal Extremity Arteries with Intraarterial Injections and Digital Subtraction

In patients with impending loss of a digit or limb, the feasibility of surgical intervention must be evaluated. In many cases, this may mean a bypass graft to the smaller vessels of the extremity. Unfortunately, conventional angiography sometimes fails to demonstrate the small branches adequately. Intraarterial injections of contrast using digital subtraction have been able to better define these vessels. The contrast enhancement capability of DSA allows visualization of these distal vessels, such as the distal radial and ulnar arteries, the palmar arches and digital arteries of the hand, the anterior and posterior tibial arteries, the dorsalis pedis artery, the plantar arch, and the plantar and digital arteries of the foot. Visualization of the anterior and posterior tibial arteries may be most important since these are potential sites for bypass grafts (Fig. 8-14). If the smallest distal vessels of an extremity are occluded, such as the arteries of the hand or foot, surgical intervention is not technically feasible at this time. In Figure 8-15, a patient with Raynaud's phenomenon and threatened loss of a digit is shown. The arteries were occluded at a level that prevented surgical intervention.

EXPECTATIONS FOR THE FUTURE

Safety, cost, and accuracy have already resulted in the use of intravenous angiography for screening of the renal arteries in hypertensive patients.[4] Digital subtraction angiograms of the carotid arteries are now performed even in patients with minimal symptomatoiogy.

Under development is a very large high-resolution prototype image intensifier with a diameter of 22 inches (Siemens, Phoenix, AZ). If used for peripheral angiography, it would allow complete evaluation with only two or three runs, and would

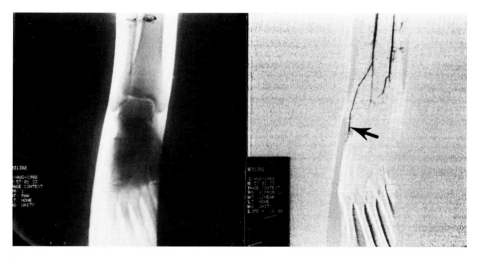

Figure 8-15. The raw data frame and an intraarterial digital subtraction angiogram of the right foot demonstrates complete occlusion of the posterior and anterior tibial arteries at the level of the malleoli. Only one small vessel is seen supplying any part of the foot (arrow). Vascular reconstruction was not possible. The patient had Raynaud's phenomenon.

require a volume of contrast similar to that now used for conventional angiograms. Such a unit could conceivably permit the use of DSA for screening patients with suspected vascular occlusive disease.

REFERENCES

1. Sigstedt B, Lunderquist A: Complications of angiographic examinations. AJR 130:455–460, 1978
2. Greenstone SM, Massell TB, Heringman EC: Hazards and complications of retrograde aortography and arteriography. Angiology 16:93–98, 1965
3. Detmer DE, Fryback DG, Strother CM: Digital subtraction arteriography cost-effectiveness, in Mistretta CA, Crummy AB, Strothers CM, et al (eds): Digital Subtraction Arteriography. Chicago, Year Book, 1982
4. Hillman BJ, Ovitt TW, Capp MP, et al: The potential impact of digital video subtraction angiography on screening for renovascular hypertension. Radiology 142:577–579, 1982
5. Dempsey PJ, Goree JA, Jimenez JP, et al: The effect of contrast media on patient motion during cerebral angiography. Radiology 115:207–209, 1975
6. Guthaner DF, Silverman JF, Mayden WG, et al: Intraarterial analgesia in peripheral arteriography. AJR 128:737–739, 1977
7. Pond GD, Osborne RW, Capp MP, et al: Digital subtraction angiography of peripheral vascular bypass procedures. AJR 138:279–281, 1982
8. Freedman DS: Economic analysis of outpatient digital angiography. Appl Radiol 11:29–38, 1982
9. Crummy AB, Strother CM, Liebermann RP, et al: Digital video subtraction angiography for evaluation of peripheral vascular disease. Radiology 141:33–37, 1981
10. Hillman BJ, Smith JRL, Pond GD, et al: Photoelectronic Radiology, vol 4. New York, John Wiley & Sons, 1982

Jonathan E. Hasson
Steven A. Gould
Gerald S. Moss

9

Blood Flow Laboratory Evaluation of the Veins

Deep vein thrombosis continues to be a major clinical problem because the condition may lead to two significant sequelae: pulmonary embolism, and postphlebitic syndrome. Pulmonary embolism remains one of the chief causes of morbidity and mortality in hospitalized patients and is the major acute risk of deep vein thrombosis. The late consequence of deep vein thrombosis is the so-called postphlebitic syndrome, which is a result of the destruction of the valves in the deep venous system and the resultant chronic venous insufficiency. The swelling, discomfort, and eventual ulceration associated with this entity are often the cause of chronic debilitation.

An early and accurate diagnosis of acute deep vein thrombosis is necessary for adequate therapy. With early diagnosis, effective anticoagulant therapy can be instituted before major embolism occurs, and unnecessary therapy with its attendant risks can be avoided. Early therapy may also be helpful in minimizing damage to the deep venous valves, so that long-term morbidity might be decreased. Finally, patients with an established diagnosis of chronic venous insufficiency and recurrent symptoms are often inappropriately treated with repeated hospitalization and prolonged anticoagulation. A simple and accurate test for the diagnosis of both acute deep vein thrombosis and chronic venous insufficiency is important if inappropriate diagnosis and therapy are to be avoided.

A diagnosis of deep vein thrombosis made solely on the basis of classical physical findings (tenderness, swelling, Homans' sign) is highly inaccurate;[1] at best, the correlation between physical findings and contrast phlebography is 50 percent. The associated risks of phlebography;[2] performed on a routine basis include a 6 percent incidence of dye-induced allergic reactions. In one study,[3] 18 percent of contrast phlebograms inadequately visualized the common femoral and iliac systems, and Strandness[2] has reported inadequate visualization of the deep femoral system in as many as 50 percent of studies. In addition, contrast phlebography is somewhat painful

IMAGING OF THE PERIPHERAL VASCULAR SYSTEM Copyright © 1984 by Grune & Stratton.
ISBN   0-8089-1636-X

and occasionally difficult. These limitations have spurred the development of several noninvasive modalities for the diagnosis of deep vein thrombosis. The Doppler ultrasound examination of the venous system and various plethysmographic techniques will be discussed in this chapter.

DOPPLER EXAMINATION

Technique

The technique of examining the lower extremities with Doppler ultrasound has been well described[2-4] and will be briefly summarized here. The four major veins of the leg (the common femoral, the superficial femoral, the popliteal, and the posterior tibial at the medial malleolus) are sequentially examined. A 5-MHz Doppler probe is optimal for the examination. The veins are located by their known anatomic relations to arteries, and Doppler signals are examined for their presence, phasicity (variation with respiration), and changes with compression and release, both proximal and distal to the probe.

The femoral and posterior tibial systems are examined with the patient supine and with the patient's knee in slight flexion to eliminate possible compression of the popliteal vein as it crosses the knee. The popliteal vein is examined with the patient prone and the knee supported in slight flexion.

Briefly, the signal heard over a major vein will be perceived as a low-pitched "whooshing" sound, much akin to the sound of the wind (Fig. 9-1A). The absence of spontaneous signals signifies significant occlusion of the vein (Fig. 9-1B).

Normal venous signals will vary in intensity with respirations. (Fig. 9-1A) With inspiration, the diaphragm descends, intraabdominal pressure increases, and flow in the venous system decreases. The reverse situation is true for expiration. A Valsalva's maneuver has the expected effect of decreasing flow because of the resultant increase in venous resistance. The absence of phasic changes of the venous system with respiration suggests significant venous occlusion (Fig. 9-1B). Although collateral venous channels often have spontaneous signals, they do not, in general, exhibit normal phasic changes.

Other maneuvers, such as compression proximal or distal to the probe add additional information to the Doppler examination. Distal manual compression of the limb should produce an augmentation of the venous signal proximally (Fig. 9-1C). A decrease or absence of augmentation is suggestive of occlusion proximal to the compression site (Fig. 9-1D). Compression proximal to the probe should normally decrease or obliterate the signal (Fig. 9-1E). Release of compression proximal to the probe should then produce an augmentation of the Doppler signal (Fig. 9-1E). Absence of this response is also suggestive of significant obstruction.

Valvular incompetence may be assessed by proximal compression. In a normal extremity, with competent one-way venous valves, the flow should decrease or disappear with proximal compression (Fig. 9-1E). A to-and-fro spontaneous sound or augmentation of the signal distally during proximal compression is indicative of valvular incompetence (Fig. 9-1F).

Normal and significant positive findings are tabulated in Table 9-1.

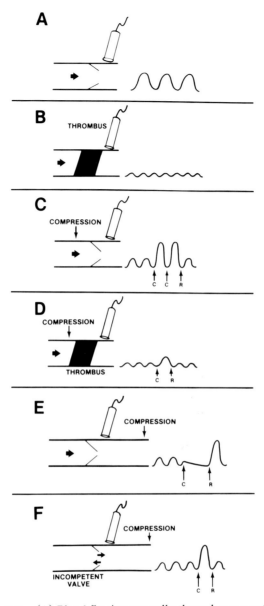

Figure 9-1. (A) Blood flowing normally through a competent valve. The Phasic signal present with respiration is shown on the right. (B) Thrombus in a vein; there is an absence of a spontaneous signal and loss of respiratory variation. (C) Distal compression (C) should augment the signal proximally. With release (R), the signal returns to baseline. (D) Thrombus prevents a significant proximal augmentation of the signal with distal compression. (E) Proximal compression (C) should obliterate the normal signal, while subsequent release will lead to an augmentation of the signal. (F) Proximal compression (C) will augment the venous signal distally with incompetent valves. Release (R) will return the signal to baseline.

Table 9-1

Normal and Significant Positive Findings on Doppler Ultrasound
Examination

	Normal	Abnormal	Diagnosis
Spontaneous signal	Present*	Absent or decreased	Occlusion
Respiratory changes	Present	Absent (continuous)	Occlusion
Distal compression proximal release	Increased signal	Absent o small change	Occlusion
Proximal compression	Decrease or absent signal	Increased signal	Incompetent valves

*May not be present in posterior tibial system.

Limitations

Several factors may affect the outcome of the venous examination. A particularly
large thigh may render the superficial femoral vein inaccessible to thorough examination. Very large collateral channels may show respiratory variation and lead to a
false-negative examination. The popliteal vein is occasionally difficult to examine and
is best found by a trained examiner. Too much pressure exerted on the probe may
obliterate a normal venous channel and produce a false-positive result. Finally, the
venous signal may be pulsatile in the presence of congestive heart failure or tricuspid
insufficiency, making results hard to interpret.

Accuracy in Diagnosis

Several authors[3-7] have shown that a carefully performed Doppler examination
of the venous system will have an accuracy rate between 85 and 95 percent in the
diagnosis of deep vein thrombosis in those patients suspected of having the disease
(when compared with contrast phlebography). The false-negative rate is variously
quoted between 2 and 15 percent. It is unlikely that significant deep vein thrombosis
is present in the face of a normal Doppler examination.[7]

A major limitation in the use of the Doppler examination is the inability to
accurately detect small, nonocclusive or isolated calf vein thrombi. Many authors,
however, are in agreement that isolated calf vein thrombi do not pose a significant
threat to the patient and may be best left untreated.[6,7,8]

As an isolated modality, the Doppler examination has been shown to be an
excellent tool for detecting the presence of deep vein thrombosis. A strongly positive
examination, or a significant change from a previously normal examination, is regarded
as an indication for the institution of anticoagulant therapy.[4,5,7,9,10] Of course, if clinical
suspicion of deep vein thrombosis remains high in the presence of a negative Doppler
study, phlebography is indicated.

The Doppler examination has proved to be a rapid, painless, portable, and easy
method for the diagnosis of deep vein thrombosis. This has allowed unnecessary

anticoagulant therapy to be avoided, and has provided a safe, practical means for screening, diagnosis, and follow-up.

PLETHYSMOGRAPHIC TECHNIQUES

Other techniques have been devised, which, when used alone or in conjunction with the Doppler examination, have improved the ability of physicians to accurately and noninvasively diagnose deep vein thrombosis. The plethysmographic techniques are designed to measure the rate of venous outflow from a limb by indirectly measuring changes in the volume (i.e., blood volume) of that limb.

Strain-Gauge Plethysmography

Strain-gauge plethysmography has been well described.[3,9,10,11] The rate of venous outflow of a limb is indirectly assessed by measuring the changes in circumference of two Silastic bands placed on the calf, while an occluding cuff in the thigh is inflated and released (Fig. 9-2).

The rate of change in limb volume is graphically represented on a strip-chart recorder. A typical normal tracing is presented in Fig. 9-3. Barnes[9] has shown that there are significant differences in the maximum rate of venous outflow (MVO) between normal limbs and limbs with acute thrombophlebitis (41 ml/min/100 ml versus 12

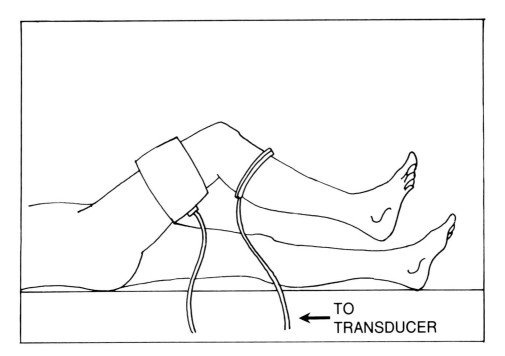

Figure 9-2. Strain-gauge plethysmography. Silastic bands are connected to the transducer. The limb between the bands is treated as a truncated cone for volume measurements.

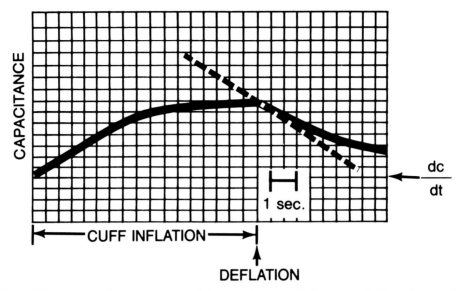

Figure 9-3. Volume changes as measured by a strain-gauge plethysmograph. A maximum rate of venous outflow (MVO) can be calculated as: $(-2/C) \times (dc/dt) \times 60 \times 100$ (ml/min/100 ml tissue in calf) where C is the calf circumference in millimeters, and dc/dt is the rate of change in calf circumference in millimeters per second.

ml/min/100 ml). It is presumed that in the presence of significant thrombosis, the venous emptying through collateral channels is slower. Strandness[2] has stated that this method is 90-percent accurate in the diagnosis of deep vein thrombosis.

Impedance Plethysmography

The impedance plethysmography (IPG), described by Wheeler et al.,[12] has become the most common noninvasive machine in use. Again, this technique attempts to measure venous outflow by quantitating changes in the electrical impedance of a limb. Since blood is a better conductor of electricity than fat and muscle, the resistance (impedance) of a limb decreases as the volume of blood in the extremity increases. By measuring changes in the impedance of a limb, the blood volume of the limb (inflow and outflow) can be indirectly assessed.

The limb to be studied is elevated, and four aluminum strips are placed on the calf. A weak high-frequency current is passed between the strips, and voltage measurements are made while a large thigh cuff is inflated and released. As the thigh cuff is inflated, the venous outflow is occluded and the limb volume increases. This is measured as a decreased impedance. With cuff release, the reverse occurs. A normal tracing is shown in Figure 9-4.

Figure 9-5 is an IPG tracing from a patient with significant deep vein thrombosis. Note the slower rate of venous outflow.

Because venous capacitance (inflow) can vary as a result of calf muscle tension and respiratory effort, both the capacitance and the rate of venous outflow (over 3 seconds) are measured multiple times. In a large study using the impedance plethysmograph, Hull et al.[13] has shown via discriminant analysis that proximal deep vein

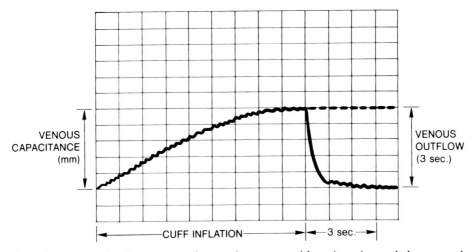

Figure 9-4. A tracing from a normal extremity as seen with an impedance plethysmograph.

thrombosis can be diagnosed with greater than 90-percent accuracy by the measurement of outflow and capacitance. Results of patients in Figures 9-4 and 9-5 are plotted on a discriminant graph in Figure 9-6. Like the Doppler examination, the effectiveness of this technique is limited in those patients with isolated calf vein thrombi and nonocclusive thrombi. The development of significant collateral channels after an episode of deep vein thrombosis may also give rise to false-negative results; therefore, this study is best performed early.

The combination of plethysmographic (strain-gauge or impedance) and Doppler examination has been shown to increase the overall accuracy of diagnosis of deep vein thrombosis to 93 to 95 percent.[7] The significance of missed isolated calf vein thrombi has been questioned. Yao et al.[7] has followed 45 patients with calf vein thrombi and

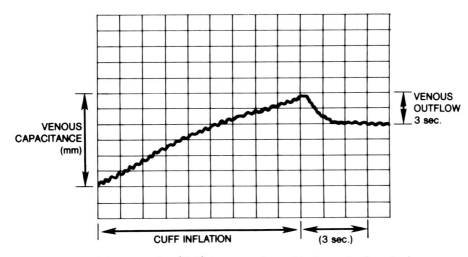

Figure 9-5. A tracing (IPG) from a patient with deep vein thrombosis.

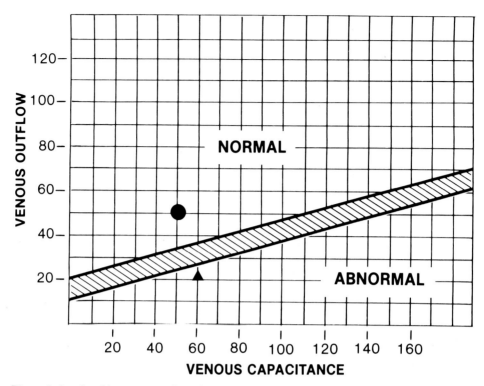

Figure 9-6. Graphic representation of 90-percent confidence limits for diagnosis of deep vein thrombosis with impedance plethysmography. The values for the patient in Figure 9-5 plotted with the triangle.

negative IPG and Doppler examinations for 2 years and has reported no additional significant venous thrombosis or pulmonary embolism in this group.

It must be remembered that these tests are indeed noninvasive, and extrinsic compression of the venous system (tumor, hematoma, Baker's cyst, lymphedema) may produce positive studies. In the presence of a phlebogram that does not reveal intrinsic defects, these and other causes of venous occlusion obviously need to be investigated. Clinical judgment cannot be omitted.

The impedance plethysmographic examination, in conjunction with Doppler examination, is a safe bedside technique that is easily performed and highly accurate in the diagnosis of major calf or proximal deep vein thrombosis. Positive results should be an indication for anticoagulation, and negative results essentially rule out proximal deep vein thrombosis. A change from a normal examination is also highly suspicious. Again, if the two tests disagree, or if clinical suspicion is high, contrast phlebography is then indicated.

Photoplethysmography

The photoplethysmograph (PPG) has become an important tool in the study of chronic venous insufficiency. This tool uses an infrared sensor to detect blood content in the skin. With PPG measurements, the "venous recovery time" of a limb may be studied.

In normal limbs, direct measurements of ankle venous pressures can be made at rest and with exercise (dorsal and plantar flexion of the feet). In a healthy limb, the venous pressure will drop during exercise (increased muscle pump activity with increased venous outflow), and return to normal in a fixed time when exercise ceases. In a limb with chronic deep vein insufficiency, the fall in pressure measured at the ankle during exercise will be less because of the presence of incompetent valves, and the time to return to pre-exercise levels (venous recovery time) will be shorter (more reflux).

The venous recovery time can be accurately and noninvasively measured by studying the microcirculation of the skin at the ankle with the PPG. This has been shown to correlate well with direct intravenous measurements.[14] Mean venous recovery time as measured by PPG was 48 seconds in normal patients. Patients with postphlebitic syndrome had average recovery times of 12 seconds.[14] The PPG technique now provides an objective way to document the presence of chronic venous insufficiency, and, in conjunction with Doppler tests for valvular reflux, will help to more accurately diagnose this disorder.

As can be seen, the noninvasive examinations (Doppler, IPG, PPG) now provide accurate means for the diagnosis of disease of the venous system. If clinical suspicion is present, and the examinations are suggestive of venous thrombosis, treatment can begin without phlebography. Figure 9-7 is a decision tree for the management of swollen legs in which deep vein thrombosis is expected.

If the PPG examination is positive (shortened venous refill time) and the patient has had previous bouts of "phlebitis," and if Doppler examinations and IPG findings are unchanged or normal, the patient may be treated for the postphlebitic syndrome.

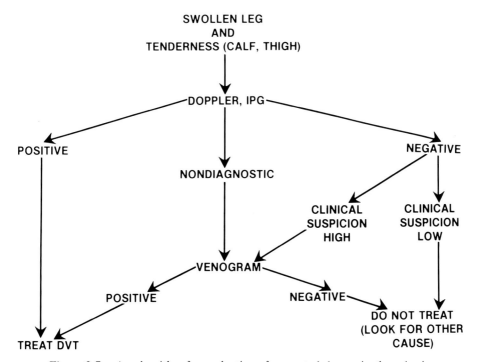

Figure 9-7. An algorithm for evaluation of suspected deep vein thrombosis.

In summary, the noninvasive techniques described represent a simple, rapid, reproducible, and accurate means of aiding in the diagnosis of acute and chronic venous disease. When properly used, the indications for the contrast venogram can be easily defined, the number of negative studies minimized, and proper treatment may be optimized.

REFERENCES

1. McLachlin J, Richard T, Paterson, JC: An evaluation of clinical signs in the diagnosis of DVT. Arch Surg 85:738–744, 1962

2. Strandness DE Jr: Invasive and noninvasive techniques in the detection and evaluation of acute venous thrombosis. Vasc Surg 11:205, 1977

3. Yao JST, Gourmos C, Hobbs JJ: Detection of proximal vein thrombosis of Doppler ultrasound flow detection method. Lancet 1:1–4, 1972

4. Strandness DE Jr, Sumner DS: Ultrasonic velocity detector in the diagnosis of thrombophlebitis. Arch Surg 104:118–183, 1972

5. Barnes RW, Russell HE, Wu KK: Accuracy of Doppler ultrasound in clinically suspected venous thrombosis of the calf. Surg Gynecol Obstet 143:425–428, 1976

6. Sumner DS, Lambeth A: Reliability of Doppler ultrasound in the diagnosis of acute venous thrombosis both above and below the knee. Am J Surg 138:205–210, 1979

7. Yao JST, Henkin RE, Bergan JJ: Venous thromboembolic disease. Arch Surg 109:664–670, 1974

8. Kakkar VV, Howe CT: Natural history of postoperative deep vein thrombosis. Lancet 2:230–233, 1969

9. Barnes RW, Collicott PE, Mozersky DJ, et al: Noninvasive quantitation of maximum venous outflow in acute thrombophlebitis. Surgery 72:971–979, 1972

10. Johnson WC: Evaluation of newer techniques for the diagnosis of venous thrombosis. J Surg Res 16:473–481, 1974

11. Nicholas GG, Miller FJ, Demith WE, et al: Clinical vascular laboratory diagnosis of deep venous thrombosis. Ann Surg 186:213–215, 1977

12. Wheeler HB, Pearson D, O'Connell D, et al: Impedance phlebography: Technique, interpretation and results. Arch Surg 104:164–169, 1972

13. Hull R, Van Aken WG, Hirsh J, et al: Impedance plethysmography using the occlusive cuff technique in the diagnosis of venous thrombosis. Circulation 53:696–700, 1976

14. Abramowitz HB, Queral LA, Flinn WR, et al: The use of photoplethysmography in the assessment of venous insufficiency: A comparison to venous pressure measurements. Surgery 86:434–441, 1979

Carlos Bekerman

10

The Fibrinogen Uptake Test and Fibrinogen Scintigraphy for Detection of Deep Vein Thrombosis

Thromboembolism is recognized as a major hazard to life. It has been estimated that in the United States close to 50,000 patients die of pulmonary embolic disease each year. Primarily, these are mothers in childbirth or patients who have undergone surgery. The major cause of pulmonary embolism is venous thrombosis of the lower extremities or pelvis. Pulmonary embolism is also a common complication in prostrating medical illnesses. When not fatal, deep vein thrombosis may produce extensive local damage of the venous valves, with the sequelae of varicose veins, swelling of the legs, or persistent pain.[1] Accurate recognition of this disorder at an early stage is not easy because of the lack of specificity of its clinical manifestations.

The development of new, sensitive, specific, and noninvasive techniques has led to more accurate diagnosis of deep vein thrombosis and to effective evaluation of its response to therapy. The ^{125}I-fibrinogen uptake test (^{125}I-FUT) and ^{123}I-fibrinogen scintigraphy are two of these new techniques. The use of each of these tests, as well as their advantages, indications, and limitations in the diagnosis of venous thrombosis will be discussed.

FIBRINOGEN UPTAKE TEST

Radiopharmaceutical: Preparation, Labeling, Dose and Administration

Animal experiments have demonstrated preferential uptake of ^{131}I-fibrinogen by a forming thrombus.[2] The first clinical experience with the use of ^{131}I-labeled fibrinogen in the detection of deep vein thrombosis was reported by Palko et al.[3] in 1964. However, the many disadvantages of ^{131}I as a label for fibrinogen led to its replacement by ^{125}I.[4]

For the ^{125}I-FUT, either autologous or homologous fibrinogen that has been separated from plasma are used. The risk of serum hepatitis is eliminated when autologous fibrinogen is used; however, autologous fibrinogen is not practical for routine use. Careful screening of donors eliminates the risk of hepatitis and thus allows the use of homologous fibrinogen, which is preferable.

Iodine-125 is the label of choice for the FUT because it has a conveniently long half-life (60 days), which allows monitoring of thrombi over extended periods. Several methods for labeling of fibrinogen with ^{125}I are available.[5] One or two atoms of iodine per molecule of fibrinogen are sufficient. The unbound radioiodine remaining after radioiodination is removed.

Approximately 1 mg of fibrinogen labeled with 100 μCi of ^{125}I is administered to the patient intravenously. This activity is sufficient for monitoring of the patient for 1 to 2 weeks.

The high tissue absorption of ^{125}I because of its low-energy gamma radiation (35 keV) limits the detectable surface counts. For this reason, imaging is not possible with currently available instruments.

Dosimetry

Replacement of ^{131}I by ^{125}I has drastically reduced the total-body radiation dose to the patient. Following the injection of 100 μCi of ^{125}I fibrinogen, the total-body radiation has been estimated at between 100 and 200 mrem.[6] Free radioiodine in the preparation accounts for a somewhat higher dose to the thyroid gland and other iodine-concentrating organs. The radiation dose to the thyroid gland is reduced markedly by oral administration of 1 ml (20 drops) of stable iodide (Lugol's solution) approximately 24 hours before the radiopharmaceutical is administered, and once a day while the patient is being monitored. Sodium or potassium perchlorate may be given in place of Lugol's solution to patients who are sensitive to iodine.

Although ^{125}I-fibrinogen does not cross the placenta, the small quantities of free ^{125}I present can do so. Iodine-125 has also been found in the milk of lactating women.[7]

Method of Detection

The instrument used for counting is a light-weight, hand-held portable detector designed specifically for use with ^{125}I-fibrinogen. It has a sodium iodide crystal 1 to 1.5 cm in diameter and 1 to 2 mm thick. A scaler or a rate meter measures the radioactivity.

Before initial counting, marks are made over the patient's precordium and on the legs (Fig. 10-1). The legs are marked sequentially in 2-inch segments starting from the inguinal ligament along the medial thigh, following the course of the femoral vein to the medial border of the popliteal area, and from the posterior popliteal area along the dorsal aspect of the calf downward to the ankle.

The patient should empty the urinary bladder before counting so that falsely high counts in the proximal thigh areas caused by accumulation of radioactive iodine in the urinary bladder are avoided. The patient is monitored while supine in bed. The legs are elevated to 15 to 20 degrees above the level of the heart for at least 5 minutes before counting; this decreases venous pooling of blood and allows access of the

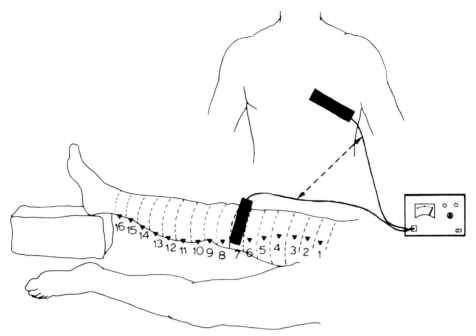

Figure 10-1. Iodine-125-fibrinogen uptake test. A portable detector-rate meter is used for measurement of the count rate over both the heart and the veins of the leg. Before measurement of the count rate in the lower extremity, the leg is elevated for at least 5 minutes so that the veins are emptied. [Reprinted from De Nardo SJ: Role of nuclear medicine in the detection of venous thrombosis, in Freeman LM, Weissman HS (Eds): New York, Raven Press, 1980, p 341. With permission.]

counter to the calf. Sites of trauma, surgery, or any disease in the lower extremities are noted.

Counts over each of the segments marked on the legs are obtained and are divided by the counts over the precordium, which are taken as 100 percent. In this way, a leg-to-heart ratio or index is obtained. Measurements at 1 hour and 4 hours after injection are advisable when active disease is suspected. Counting is done daily for 1 week, or until the test is positive. The patient's body background counts before injection and the room activity during each counting session should also be recorded.

Interpretation, Indications, and Limitations

A uniform procedure for counting should be followed precisely so that reproducible data are obtained.[8-10] The typical pattern in a normal study consists of a gradual decrease in activity from the inguinal ligament down to the ankle, with a slight increase at the back of the knee.

An ^{125}I-FUT is considered positive when there is a difference in uptake in the same site on the opposite leg (criterion 1), a difference in uptake in adjacent sites on the same leg (criterion 2), or a change in activity compared with uptake measured earlier over the same site (criterion 3) (Fig. 10-2). A difference of 20 percent in uptake is used as a threshhold level for abnormality. Abnormalities are confirmed if the

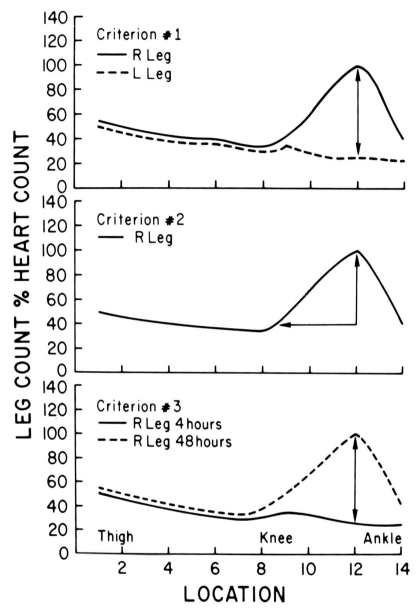

Figure 10-2. Criteria for a positive ^{125}I-fibrinogen uptake test. Criterion 1: Difference in uptake compared with that in same site on the opposite side. Criterion 2: Difference in uptake between adjacent areas on the same leg. Criterion 3: Change in uptake in the same area over time. Any one of these is a criterion for a positive study. [Reprinted from De Nardo GL, De Nardo SI, Barnett CA, et al: Assessment of conventional criteria for the early diagnosis of thrombophlebitis with the 125-I-fibrinogen uptake test. Radiology 125:765, 1977. With permission.]

increased counts persist during the subsequent 24 hours. A study is considered positive if any one of the three criteria applies.

The ^{125}I-FUT has several clinical applications. It can document established venous thrombosis. As reported by De Nardo et al.,[8-13] it can also provide early evidence of active thrombosis. At least one criterion for positivity may be present in two thirds of patients with existing thrombophlebitis as early as 3 to 4 hours after injection of ^{125}I-fibrinogen. Ninety-eight percent of patients may meet one or more criteria for abnormality by 24 hours after injection.

The overall sensitivity and specificity of the test for venous thrombosis are approximately 90 percent.[6] However, the sensitivity varies with the location of the thrombi and with their age. The ^{125}I-FUT has a higher sensitivity for the detection of thrombi in calf veins than for those in veins of the upper third of the thigh. Furthermore, in the calf vein area the ^{125}I-FUT is a more sensitive test than is contrast venography. The test is less satisfactory for the detection of thrombi in the pelvic veins because radioactive iodine accumulates in the bladder, and because the weak emissions of ^{125}I are attenuated by the tissue mass of the pelvic area.

If possible, contrast venography should not be performed before the ^{125}I-FUT, since venous thrombosis caused by the resulting inflammation of the vein wall makes the interpretation of the ^{125}I-FUT difficult.

The ^{125}I-FUT is indicated for prospective studies, particularly in surgical patients; it is also an accurate and reliable method for detection of thrombophlebitis in patients with fractures of the femoral head.[14] The test is useful as a means for following the course of venous thrombosis, for measuring the effect of treatment, and for investigating the efficacy of preventive methods.[12]

Careful clinical examination of the legs is necessary so that patients who have pathologic conditions associated with fibrinogen deposition (e.g., severe edema, symptomatic arthritis, cellulitis, hematoma, pronounced varicose veins, injections, or surgery) can be excluded. If the ^{125}I-FUT is clinically indicated, however, reliable results may be obtained if areas of the legs that contain such abnormalities are avoided. The accuracy of the ^{125}I-FUT is not affected by heparin or by warfarin given for less than 6 days.[15]

FIBRINOGEN SCINTIGRAPHY

The limitations of the ^{125}I-FUT have led to the search for radionuclides for the labeling of fibrinogen that will allow the spatial distribution of radioactivity to be imaged and the entire body or the lower part of the trunk and extremities to be surveyed for areas of increased protein deposition. At the same time, the test should help to separate the round areas of abnormal uptake in patients with arthritis and hematomas from the uptake along vascular structures.

Imaging of intracardiac and venous thrombi with ^{131}I-labeled antibodies to fibrinogen was first reported by Spar et al.[16] Charkes et al.[17] performed whole-body scintiscans in patients who had received ^{131}I-fibrinogen and found 93-percent agreement with the results of radiopaque venography. De Nardo et al.[18] were the first to report on the use of ^{123}I-fibrinogen for imaging of thrombi in dogs and subsequently in humans.

Radiopharmaceutical: Preparation, Labeling, Dose, and Administration

As for the ^{125}I-FUT, homologous fibrinogen is obtained from carefully selected hepatitis-free donors, and the fibrinogen is labeled with radioactive iodine.[5] De Nardo et al.[19] use overiodinated fibrinogen (40 iodine atoms per molecule of fibrinogen) for their clinical fibrinogen imaging studies. The disadvantages of ^{125}I as a label were noted earlier.

Iodine-131 is a radionuclide that emits photons of different energies that degrade the spatial resolution. The prolonged biologic half-life of ^{131}I-labeled fibrinogen limits the amount of activity that can be administered. The dose must be restricted to several hundred microcuries, resulting in a limited photon flux and a lengthy imaging procedure. Furthermore, the beta emission of ^{131}I results in a substantial radiation burden to the patient. Iodine-123 is the label of choice for fibrinogen scintigraphy because it emits 159-keV monoenergetic photons, which makes it ideal for imaging. It has a half-life of 13.3 hours and has no beta emissions. Technetium-99m has also been used for labeling of fibrinogen, but it has been difficult to obtain a clinically useful compound.[20-22] Approximately 1 to 2 mg of fibrinogen labeled with 1.5 to 4 mCi of ^{123}I is administered intravenously.

The uptake of ^{123}I by the thyroid can be blocked if the patient is given 1 ml of Lugol's solution (about 20 drops) approximately 24 hours before the injection of the radiopharmaceutical.

Dosimetry

The whole-body radiation dose delivered by ^{123}I-labeled fibrinogen is significantly less than that delivered by ^{125}I or [131]I. One millicurie of ^{123}I delivers 25 mrad to the whole body, whereas, for the same dose, ^{131}I delivers a whole-body dose of 1000 mrad, and [125]I a dose of 100 mrad.

Method of Detection

Imaging can be performed with a scintillation camera and a moving table for whole-body scanning. A low-energy, high-sensitivity parallel-hole collimator is used. The imaging conditions are set up and an information density of at least 700 counts/cm^2 is obtained from an initial measurement of the count rate over the pelvis with the bladder empty.

Interpretation, Indications, and Limitations

The normal and abnormal patterns of the ^{123}I-fibrinogen body distribution have been described in detail by De Nardo et al.[23] Figure 10-3 shows the normal distribution 1 day after injection. The heart, major vessels, liver, spleen, and kidneys are visualized because they contain large intravascular spaces. Activity in the veins is most notable in the iliofemoral system and gradually decreases centripetally. The thyroid and salivary glands may be visualized if they have not been properly blocked. Unbound ^{123}I may be seen in the bladder.

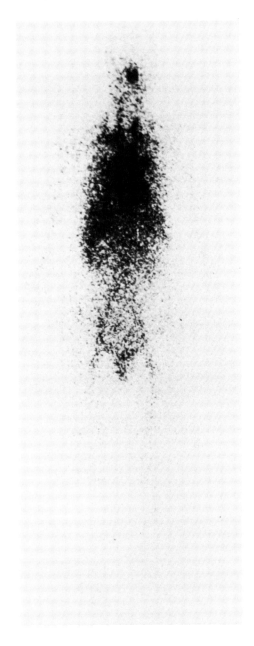

Figure 10-3. Normal pattern of distribution (intravascular and extracellular) of ^{123}I-fibrinogen at 24 hours. The heart, major vessels, liver, spleen, and kidneys, as well as paranasal and vaginal areas are visualized. Activity in veins gradually decreases centripetally and is most notable in the iliofemoral system. No unbound ^{123}I is present in the thyroid or bladder of this female patient. [Reprinted from De Nardo SJ, De Nardo GL: Iodine-123-fibrinogen scintigraphy. Semin Nucl Med 7:245, 1977. With permission.]

Five distinctive patterns of abnormal ^{123}I-fibrinogen distribution have been found that provide evidence for thrombophlebitis: (1) Centrifugal increase in the amount of radioactivity along the venous system despite diminution in the size of the vein; (2) asymmetry of distribution of radioactivity in the venous system; (3) abrupt termination of radioactivity within a vein; (4) irregular distribution (beading pattern) of radioactivity within a vein; and (5) visualization of collateral veins, particularly in the lateral aspect of the thigh and pelvis (Fig. 10-4).

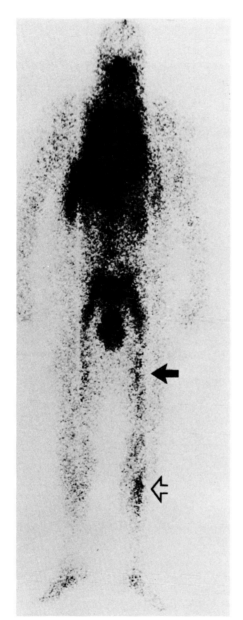

Figure 10-4. Thrombophlebitis of the venous system of both lower extremities, extending from the iliac veins to the veins of the lower calf. An irregular pattern is present in the left femoral vein (solid arrow). Asymmetric and centripetal patterns are visible in the left calf (open arrow). Radioactivity is present in the genitourinary system, heart, liver, lungs, and paranasal sinuses. [Reprinted from De Nardo SJ, De Nardo GL: Iodine-123-fibrinogen scintigraphy. Semin Nucl Med 7:245, 1977. With permission.]

De Nardo et al.[23] have found a unilateral increase of ^{123}I-fibrinogen deposition to be the most frequent and easily perceived abnormality, whereas the beading pattern is helpful in the detection of disease in the pelvic area.

Extensive pelvic or femoral thrombophlebitis with obstruction of major veins is usually associated with collateral-vein uptake. Abrupt termination of ^{123}I-fibrinogen activity suggests complete or almost complete venous obstruction.

Thrombophlebitis in the pelvis, arms, and legs may be detected readily by total-body imaging with ^{123}I-fibrinogen. According to De Nardo et al.,[24] ^{123}I-fibrinogen scintigraphy is a sensitive and specific examination for venous thrombi. In a regional comparative study of ^{123}I-fibrinogen scintigraphy and radiopaque venography, which was used as the standard, the ^{123}I-fibrinogen scintigraphic examination had 93 percent sensitivity and 89 percent specificity for the legs, and 92 percent sensitivity and 89 percent specificity by anatomic areas. No abnormal deposition of ^{123}I-fibrinogen was noted in fibrosed residual scars and dilated veins seen in radiopaque venograms.

In patients with thrombophlebitis who have received anticoagulant treatment, the findings in ^{123}I-fibrinogen scintigraphy remain positive for several days. Therefore, this test may be used for monitoring the efficacy of anticoagulant therapy, and, because of the low radiation dose, it can be repeated several times for follow-up studies of the therapeutic results. The risk of recurrent thrombophlebitis or pulmonary embolus is greater if incorporation of ^{123}I-fibrinogen persists after administration of heparin or of crystalline warfarin sodium for 10 days (Coumadin, Endo Laboratories, Wilmington, Del) for more than 1 month.

Hematomas and other conditions associated with increased deposition of fibrinogen can readily be differentiated from thrombophlebitis thanks to the spatial resolution made possible by scintigraphy.

The slow blood clearance of ^{123}I-fibrinogen makes 4-to-6 hour postinjection scintiscans more difficult to interpret than those obtained at 16 to 24 hours. The use of overiodinated fibrinogen, which continues to localize in thrombi despite being cleared rapidly from the blood, allows for an increased target-to-nontarget ratio (clot/blood), thus facilitating the interpretation of the test, particularly at early times after injection.

According to De Nardo et al.,[23] studies performed 6 hours after injection can usually be clearly interpreted as normal or abnormal. Borderline studies call for repeat imaging at 24 hours after injection, when the previously minimal clot-to-background uptake may be enhanced.

In a review of the role of nuclear medicine in the detection of venous thrombosis, De Nardo[10] concludes that the approach used in the diagnostic evaluation of a patient for thrombophlebitis should depend on the clinical situation. Radioisotope venography performed at the time of a perfusion lung scan should be done more frequently in patients hospitalized with symptoms suggestive of pulmonary emboli. This approach is probably most useful in those patients who already have lung disease, and in whom a difficult lung scan interpretation is therefore anticipated.

For patients who are at high risk of developing thrombophlebitis and in whom prospective studies are more indicated than low-dose heparin therapy, the ^{125}I-FUT is the optimal study. Ambulatory patients with minimal but worrisome symptoms may also benefit from the use of ^{125}I-FUT. However, probably the most thorough examination for thrombophlebitis is accomplished by ^{123}I-fibrinogen scintigraphy. This test is a noninvasive, simple, sensitive, and specific method, and it permits easy follow-up for observation of the response to treatment.

REFERENCES

1. Coon WW, Coller FD: Clinicopathologic correlation in thromboembolism. Surg Gynecol Obstet 109:259–269, 1957
2. Hobb JT, Davies JWL: Detection of venous thrombosis with ^{131}I-labeled fibrinogen in the rabbit. Lancet ii 2:134, 1960
3. Palko PD, Mansen EM, Fedoruk SO: The early detection of deep vein thrombosis using

[131]I-tagged human fibrinogen. Can J Surg 7:215, 1964

4. Atkins P, Hawkins LA: Detection of venous thrombosis in the legs. Lancet 2:1216–1219, 1965

5. De Nardo SJ, Jansholt AL: Iodinated fibrinogen in the detection of venous thrombosis, in Berman DS, Mason DT (eds): Clinical Nuclear Cardiology. New York, Grune & Stratton, 1981, pp 348–364

6. Kakkar VU: Fibrinogen uptake test for detection of deep vein thrombosis—a review of current practice. Semin Nucl Med 7:229–244, 1977

7. Friend JR, Kakkar VV: The diagnosis of deep vein thrombosis in the puerperium. J Obstet Gynecol Br Commonwealth 77:820–823, 1970

8. De Nardo GL, De Nardo SJ, Barnett CA, et al: Assessment of conventional criteria for the early diagnosis of thrombophlebitis with the ^{125}I-fibrinogen uptake test. Radiology 125:765–768, 1977

9. De Nardo GL, De Nardo SJ: Diagnosis of Thrombophlebitis. Medical Monograph. Arlington Heights, Ill, Amersham Corp., 1978

10. De Nardo SJ: Role of nuclear medicine in the detection of venous thrombosis, in Freeman LM, Weissman HS (eds): Nuclear Medicine Annual 1980. New York, Raven Press, 1980, pp 341–366

11. De Nardo GL, De Nardo SJ: Thrombosis detection: Fibrinogen counting and radionuclide venography. Clin Nucl Med 10S:37–45, 1981

12. De Nardo GL, and De Nardo SJ: Venous disease detection, in Greenfield LD, Uszler JM (eds): Nuclear Medicine in Clinical Practice: Selective Correlation with Ultrasound and Computerized Tomography. Deerfield Beach, Fla, International Inc., 1982, pp 141–158

13. Carretta RF, De Nardo SJ, De Nardo GL, et al: Early diagnosis of venous thrombosis

using I-125 fibrinogen. J Nucl Med 18:5–10, 1977

14. Harris WH, Salzman EW, Athanasoulis C, et al: Comparison of ^{125}I-fibrinogen count scanning with phlebography for detection of venous thrombi after elective hip surgery. N Engl J Med 292:665–667, 1975

15. Browse NL, Clapham WF, Croft AN, et al: Diagnosis of established deep vein thrombosis with the ^{125}I-fibrinogen uptake test. Br Med J 4:325–328, 1971

16. Spar IL, Varon MI, Good P, et al: Isotopic detection of thrombi. Arch Surg 92:752–758, 1966

17. Charkes ND, Dugan MA, Maier WP, et al: Scintigraphic detection of deep vein thrombosis with I-131-fibrinogen. J Nucl Med 15:1163–1165, 1974

18. De Nardo SJ, De Nardo GL, O'Brien T, et al: I-123-fibrinogen imaging of thrombi in dogs. J Nucl Med 15:487, 1974

19. De Nardo GL, Krohn KA, De Nardo SJ: Comparison of oncophilic radiopharmaceuticals, *I-fibrinogen, ^{67}Ga-citrate, ^{111}In bleomycin and *I-bleomycin in tumor-bearing mice. Cancer 40:2923–2929, 1977

20. Hale TI, Jucker A: ^{99m}Tc-fibrinogen as a thrombus-imaging agent. Br J Radiol 51(602):139–140, 1978

21. Harwig JF, Harwig SSL, Wells LD, et al: Preparation and in vitro properties of ^{99m}Tc-fibrinogen. Int J Appl Radiat Isot 27:5, 1976

22. Jeghers O, Abramovici J, Jonckheer M, et al: A chemical method for the labeling of fibrinogen with [99m]Tc. Eur J Nucl Med 3:95, 1978

23. De Nardo SJ, De Nardo GL: Iodine-123-fibrinogen scintigraphy, Semin Nucl Med 7:245–252, 1977

24. De Nardo SJ, Bogren HG, De Nardo GL: Regional comparison of I-123-fibrinogen scintigraphy (SV) and radio-opaque venography (RV) in thrombophlebitis (TP). J Nucl Med 20:633, 1979

U. Yun Ryo

11

Radionuclide Venography

The number of patients who suffer from thromboembolic disease every year is not precisely known. It is estimated that the incidence of deep vein thrombosis in the United States is about 2.5 million cases, and the consequent development of acute pulmonary embolism is estimated at over 600,000 cases every year.[1,2] Although clinical signs and symptoms of venous thrombosis are well defined in the literature, it is documented that clinical diagnosis of venous thrombosis is most unreliable.[3,4]

In 1938, Dos Santos[5] described the practical technique for contrast phlebography, and the technique remains today as the "golden standard" procedure for the diagnosis of venous thrombosis.

If contrast phlebography had been simpler and noninvasive, many noninvasive procedures for the detection of venous thrombosis would not have been developed in the last 2 decades. The difficulties with contrast phlebography are that it is invasive; it requires a skilled team; the procedure is difficult to perform in patients who do not have suitable superficial veins; and the incidence of complications such as postphlebography phlebitis, extravasation of contrast medium, or hypersensitive reactions to the contrast medium, are relatively high.[6,7]

Because of the limitations of contrast phlebography, a variety of noninvasive procedures have been developed. Noninvasive procedures currently available for the detection of venous thrombosis include: the radioiodinated fibrinogen test; radionuclide venography; ultrasonic (Doppler) studies; plethysmography; and thermography. Radionuclide venography is a simple, noninvasive, yet reliable technique for the detection of venous thrombosis.

RADIOPHARMACEUTICALS

The basic mechanism of radionuclide venography is the imaging of flow abnormalities as evidence of venous obstruction. Therefore, any radiopharmaceutical can be used to obtain images of abnormalities in the venous flow. Technetium-99m-

IMAGING OF THE PERIPHERAL VASCULAR SYSTEM Copyright © 1984 by Grune & Stratton.
ISBN 0-8089-1636-X

macroaggregated albumin (MAA) or ^{99m}Tc-albumin microspheres (MS) are currently the radiopharmaceuticals of choice, because a perfusion lung scan can be taken after the venogram without additional injection, and the labeled particles are all trapped in the lung. They thus cause no background activity in a later phase venogram.

Technetium-99m pertechnetate has been used by some investigators for radionuclide venography.[8] Obstructions of the deep veins with collateral channels can be visualized readily when venograms are properly performed during the initial flow phase of the radionuclide. Such diffusible agents, i.e., ^{99m}Tc-labeled chelating agents, technically can be used if venography is to be followed by renal or brain scintigraphy without flow studies. Such radiopharmaceuticals, however, are not the preferred agents for routine radionuclide venography.

Technetium-99m-sulfur colloid, the reticuloendothelial system imaging agent, also has been used effectively by some investigators for radionuclide venography. The authors not only demonstrated venous occlusive disease using the radiopharmaceutical, but also showed possible "tagging" of venous thrombi.[9] However, there is not enough data indicating the usefulness of this agent for venography.

The macroaggregated albumin particle was successfully labeled with ^{99m}Tc-pertechnetate by Stern et al. in 1965[10] and was effectively used for lung scanning by Gwyther and Field in 1966.[11] The first successful radionuclide venography with ^{99m}Tc-MAA was reported by Webber and his colleagues in 1969[12] and by Rosenthal and Greyson in 1970.[13]

Since 1971, both albumin microspheres and MAA have been available as commercial kits that allow instant labeling with ^{99m}Tc-pertechnetate. The entire labeling procedure (introduction of ^{99m}Tc-pertechnetate into the vial and 10 minutes of tagging time at room temperature) takes less than 15 minutes. The kit vial contains 0.3–5.0 mg of albumin particles and a 0.1–0.27 mg dose of stannous chloride or tartrate as a reducing agent, depending on the manufacturer. The amount of ^{99m}Tc-pertechnetate used to label the particles ranges from 20 to 50 mCi per vial. When the particles are labeled and left standing for over an hour, they should be resuspended by gently agitating the vial before injection. There appear to be no significant differences between MAA and MS as an imaging agent for venous abnormalities.[14]

RADIATION ABSORBED DOSE

The radiation absorbed dose from radionuclide venography is equal to the radiation dose from perfusion lung scanning. All the labeled particles are eventually trapped by the lungs, except in patients who have right-to-left intracardiac shunts. Thus, the critical organ is the lung.

Microspheres are harder than MAA because of differences in the manufacturing process and higher heating. Therefore, the biologic half-life of MS in the lung is longer than that of MAA, which produces a slightly higher radiation dose. The radiation absorbed dose from an intravenous ^{99m}Tc-labeled albumin particle is 0.2 rad/mCi to the lungs and 0.008 rad/mCi to the whole body for ^{99m}Tc-MAA, and 0.4 rad/mCi to the lungs and 0.04 rad/mCi to the whole body for ^{99m}Tc-albumin microspheres.

RADIONUCLIDE VENOGRAPHY: CLINICAL UTILIZATION

Radionuclide venography with ^{99m}Tc-labeled albumin particles was introduced in 1969 by Webber et al.[12] as a simple and reliable method for detection of thrombophlebitis. Further observations were made by Rosenthal and Greyson in 1970.[13] The advantages of this technique are (1) it is technically simple and can be performed in conjunction with the perfusion lung scan; (2) simultaneous images of the inferior vena cava, iliac veins, and femoral veins, as well as the calf veins, can be obtained with a single injection; (3) no significant complications have been reported; (4) it is suitable as a screening test for hospitalized and nonhospitalized patients; and (5) the procedure takes less than 30 minutes, and the results are available immediately.

The reliability of radionuclide venography in the detection of venous thrombosis has been repeatedly reported to be excellent.[15–24] Earlier studies, however, demonstrated considerable discrepancy between the findings of radionuclide venograms and contrast venograms at the site of the thrombosis or calf vein abnormality.[13,17,22] Recent studies on the mechanism of abnormalities in radionuclide venography indicate that venous thrombosis causes an area of decreased radioactivity flow corresponding to the region of thrombosis, abnormal collateral flows, and stasis of radioactivity below the region of thrombosis.[19,20]

PROCEDURE

Venography of the Lower Extremities

Lower extremity venography is indicated for the detection of the source and extent of venous thrombosis in patients with documented, recurrent pulmonary embolism; for the evaluation of leg veins in patients with signs and symptoms of deep vein thrombosis; in patients who are referred to the nuclear medicine department for a perfusion lung scan and who have had a recent episode of pulmonary embolism or belong to the high risk group for leg vein thrombosis; for a follow-up evaluation of the efficacy of treatment in patients with documented, extensive leg vein thrombosis; and for an evaluation of previous surgical intervention, inferior vena cava umbrella, or ligation.

The instrument of choice for this procedure is the large-field-view camera (38.7 cm or larger effective field) with a low-energy parallel-hole collimator. A conventional small-field-of-view camera (25.6 cm) can be used with a diverging-hole collimator.

With the patient supine on an imaging table, two tourniquets are applied to each leg, one above the ankle and the other below the knee. Both lower legs are aligned in the field of view of the camera.

A 2-mCi dose of ^{99m}Tc-macroaggregated albumin or ^{99m}Tc-albumin microspheres is injected into the dorsal vein of each foot. When the flow of radioactivity through the deep calf veins is visualized on a persistence scope, the tourniquets over the ankles are released. Serial flow images from the calf veins and femoral veins are obtained consecutively. Immediately after the imaging of the femoral vein, the tourniquets below the knee are released simultaneously with activation of the camera, and serial scintigrams of the thighs and pelvis are obtained. Finally, additional images of both lower legs are taken.

A normal radionuclide venogram shows radioactivity flowing without interruption through the deep calf veins, the femoral veins, the saphenous veins, the iliac veins, and the inferior caval vein (Fig. 11-1).

A successful, good quality venogram depends on the application of optimum tourniquet pressure and imaging at proper sequences. If the tourniquet below the knee is applied too tightly, the flow of radioactivity can be interrupted at the level of the tourniquet. Good visualization of the saphenous system depends on the release of the

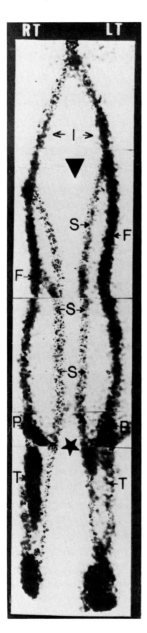

Figure 11-1. A normal radionuclide venogram of the lower extremities. When the proper sequence of the technique is followed after a simultaneous injection of ^{99m}Tc-MAA into the dorsal foot veins bilaterally, images of the major deep and superficial veins can be obtained. I = Iliac vein; S = saphenous vein; F = femoral vein; P = popliteal vein; T = tibial vein; solid triangle = region of the symphysis pubis; star = region of the knee.

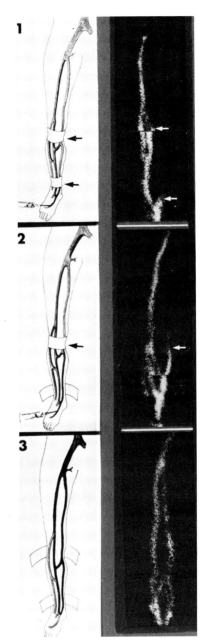

Figure 11-2. The sequence of venous flow imaging. (1) When tourniquets are applied below the knee and above the ankle and a radionuclide injection is made into a dorsal foot vein, only deep veins appear on the venogram because the flow through the superficial veins is blocked by the tourniquets (arrows). (2) Flow through the distal saphenous system can be visualized by releasing the tourniquet above the ankle (arrow). (3) Images of the entire saphenous system, in addition to the deep veins, can be made as the final step by releasing the tourniquet below the knee.

ankle tourniquet at the proper time. If the tourniquets over the ankle and below the knee are left on too long, all the radionuclide might flow through the deep veins, thus leaving an insufficient amount to flow through the saphenous system when the tourniquets are released (Fig. 11-2). Such problems can be avoided by using ^{99m}Tc-MAA mixed in a larger volume of saline, 5–10 ml, and injecting a smaller volume of the radiopharmaceutical for each view. In order to use this infusion technique, a small infusion needle must be used (e.g., a butterfly scalp vein needle). Images of all deep veins are obtained with tourniquets on, since 0.5 to 1.0 ml of the radiopharmaceutical is being injected for each view. At this point, all the tourniquets are released and images of the saphenous veins are obtained while more radiopharmaceutical is injected through the infusion needle.

Images of the entire leg vein system can be obtained on a film when a gamma camera and moving table are used[18,19] (Fig. 11-3). With a single injection technique, however, proper adjustment of the speed of the moving table will become difficult, because the speed of the flow of radioactivity (venous flow) varies with each patient.

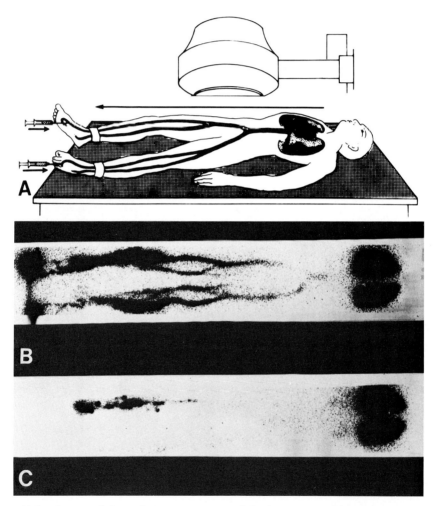

Figure 11-3. Images of the entire venous system of the lower extremities, from the ankle to the proximal inferior vena cava, including the lungs, can be imaged when the whole-body imaging system is used (see text). (A) The whole-body venogram imaging system. (B) A single-pass whole body image taken immediately after injection using a large-field-of-view camera. (C) A delayed whole-body image taken after the first images to show areas of stasis of the radionuclide.

Venography of the Upper Extremities

Radionuclide venography of the upper extremities is indicated in patients with suspected abnormalities in the deep veins of the arm and in patients who are allergic to contrast medium or patients who are undergoing a perfusion lung scan for a suspected pulmonary embolism. With the patient with suspected venous obstruction of the upper limb and a swollen arm with distended superficial veins lying supine on a imaging table, a tourniquet is applied to the middle forearm. The arm and shoulder are aligned in the field of view of the camera and a 2-mCi dose of ^{99m}Tc-MAA or ^{99m}Tc-MS is injected into the dorsal metacarpal or distal cephalic vein. After the flow of radioactivity through the subclavian vein is visualized on a persistence scope, the camera is activated and serial 20,000-count images are obtained. The tourniquet is then released and serial images are again obtained.

When areas of stasis are detected, repeat views are obtained over the area. Normal serial venograms of the upper extremity show a flow of radioactivity through the basilic vein, the brachial vein, the cephalic vein, the axillary vein, and the subclavian vein without a persistent flow defect[25] (Figs. 11-4, 11-5).

PRINCIPLES OF ABNORMAL FINDINGS

It was not until 1975 that radionuclide venography with ^{99m}Tc-albumin particles became a popular procedure, although the technique has been known since 1969.[12] One of the reasons was a controversy over the mechanism of abnormal findings. For many years, a "hot spot," or focal retention of radioactivity, was regarded as evidence of venous thrombus. If a venogram is interpreted as abnormal on the basis of the retention of radioactivity, the rate of false-positive results becomes unacceptably high. Other studies on the mechanism of positive findings of venography demonstrated that a hot spot on a venogram corresponds to stasis below the venous thrombosis.[19-21]

Radionuclide venography is a highly sensitive and reliable technique for detecting venous thrombosis when the scintigram is properly analyzed. As noted earlier, the abnormal findings consistent with venous thrombosis are an area of decreased flow corresponding to the region of thrombosis; abnormal collateral flows, and stasis of radioactivity below the region of thrombosis (Figs. 11-6, 11-7). Persistent nonvisual-

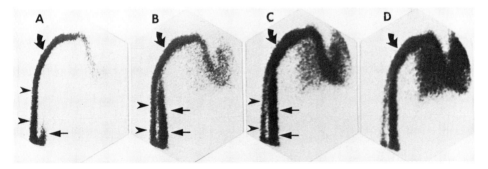

Figure 11-4. Normal upper extremity venogram. Injection of ^{99m}Tc-MAA was made into the cephalic vein above the wrist while a tourniquet was lightly applied below the elbow joint. A normal flow of radioactivity through the cephalic vein (arrow heads) into the axillary vein (curved arrow) is seen in the earliest frames (A,B). A slightly delayed flow through the brachial vein (straight arrows) is noted in the later frames (B,C,D).

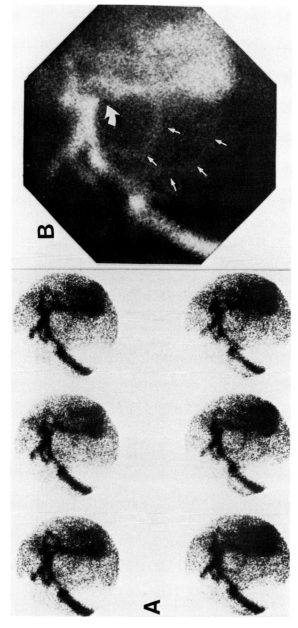

Figure 11-5. An abnormal upper extremity venogram. The flow images (A) show an area of flow interruption in the brachial vein and collateral channels. A static image (B) composed of summed flow images shows an additional flow obstruction in the bracheocephalic vein (curved arrow) and collateral flows through the superficial intercostal veins (small arrows).

218

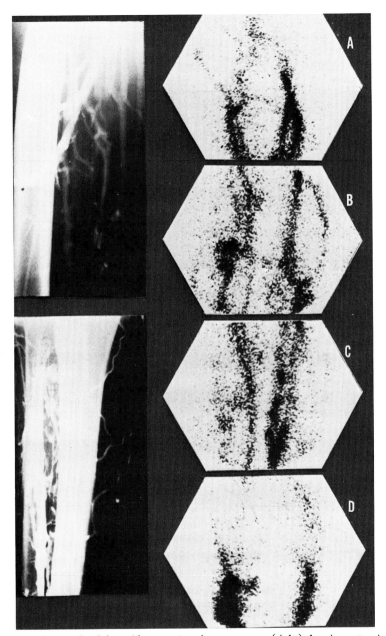

Figure 11-6. Abnormal pelvic and lower extremity venograms (right) showing extensive thrombosis in the bilateral iliac, femoral, popliteal and tibial veins. Extensive collateral channels, flow interruptions, and areas of stasis are seen. (A) Pelvic view; (B) thigh view; (C) over the knee view; (D) calf and ankle view. The extensive thrombosis was confirmed by contrast venograms (left) of the thigh and calf region.

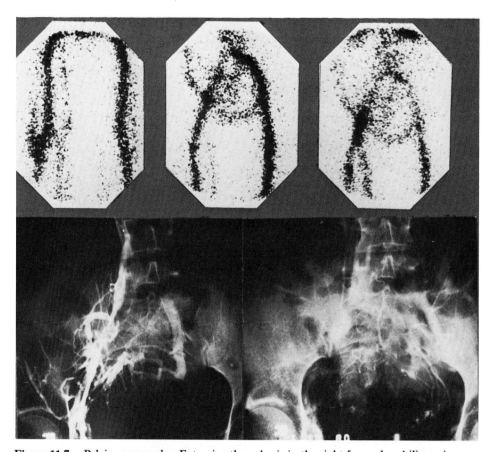

Figure 11.7. Pelvic venography. Extensive thrombosis in the right femoral and iliac veins can be noted on the venograms (top) in the form of flow interruption, collateral channels, and areas of retention of radioactivity. Occlusion of the iliac veins always causes collateral flow to the contralateral iliac vein through the pelvic venous plexus (top, middle and right). It is also common to see collateral flow through the inferior epigastric vein when there is obstruction in the iliac vein (top, middle and right). Contrast venograms of the right iliac vein (bottom) show extensive thrombosis in the right iliac vein and filling of the left iliac vein through abnormal collateral veins.

ization of a vein in serial venograms indicates obstruction of the vein as a result of thrombosis or, rarely, because of extrinsic compression. In venograms of the lower extremity, nonvisualization of either the saphenous vein or the femoral vein indicates the likelihood of thrombosis of the vein. Nonvisualization of the saphenous vein, however, can be the result of poor technique, e.g., late release of the tourniquet below the knee (Fig. 11-8). In upper extremity venography, however, the technique becomes less critical. When the injection is made through the dorsal metacarpal vein, the radioactivity should flow through all major veins of the arm unless there is thrombosis in a vein.

Stasis of radioactivity alone in the calf region on a lower extremity venogram does not represent thrombosis in the calf veins. When the finding of simple stasis in

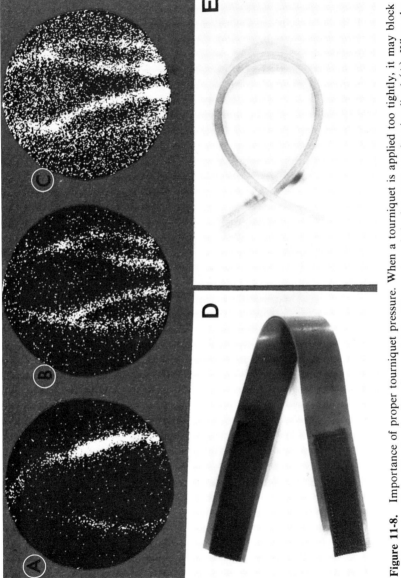

Figure 11-8. Importance of proper tourniquet pressure. When a tourniquet is applied too tightly, it may block the flow of radionuclide (venous flow) completely. Thus, veins of the leg may not be visualized (A). When the tourniquet pressure is too light or the tourniquet is released too early, most of the radioactivity may flow through the saphenous vein. Thus, the deep veins are poorly visualized or not visualized at all (C). The Venogram in (B) is correctly done. The tourniquet shown in (D) is preferred over the one shown in (E).

Table 11-1

Causes of the Abnormal Findings on Radionuclide Venograms

Abnormal Findings on Radionuclide Venogram	Number of Patients	Cause Confirmed by Contrast Venogram	Number of Patients
Persistently Cold Area	18	Thrombosis	19
Collateral Flows	22	Abnormal veins	19
		Normal branches	3
Persistently Hot Area	30	Stasis below the lesion	19
		Incompetent valve	4
		Normal valve or vein	7

Abnormal findings seen on the radionuclide venograms were correlated with the findings on contrast venograms in 50 patients on whom both procedures were performed.

the calf is regarded as nonspecific, the accuracy of venography improves significantly.[18-20] The mechanisms of abnormal findings on radionuclide venograms are summarized in Table 11-1. The reliability of radionuclide venography with ^{99m}Tc-albumin particles has been evaluated at many institutions using the results from contrast venography.

The results of agreement between radionuclide venography and contrast venography reported by various investigators are summarized in Table 11-2. It is reasonable to state that accuracy of radionuclide venography averages over 90 percent. This accuracy is superior to the average results from other noninvasive procedures for the detection of venous thrombosis.

PITFALLS IN INTERPRETING RADIONUCLIDE VENOGRAMS

A radionuclide venogram is an image of venous flow. Thus, the venogram shows a flow defect and collateral flows when there is a venous obstruction or stricture, but the image does not reveal the cause of the obstruction. This fact becomes a pitfall in

Table 11-2

Agreement between Radionuclide Venography and Contrast Venography

Authors	Accuracy* (%)
Yao JS, et al.[15]	89
Duffy GJ, et al.[22]	87
Henkins RE, et al.[16]	96
Pollack EW, et al.[17]	89
Verma RC, et al.[31]	76
Van Kirk OC, et al.[18]	95
Ryo UY, et al.[20]	89
Ennis JJ, et al.[21]	95
Hayt DB, et al.[19]	96

*Accuracy = (sensitivity + specificity) ÷ 2.

interpreting the results of the procedure, because acute thrombosis cannot be differentiated from old venous disease. Findings on the venogram also do not differentiate an intrinsic obstruction caused by thrombosis from an extrinsic obstruction, i.e., compression (Fig. 11-9 A and B). Stricture of a vein from surgical intervention is indistinguishable from abnormalities caused by thrombosis (Fig. 11-10).

Stasis of radioactivity or a "hot spot" may present difficulty in interpreting a venogram. The hot spot is a common finding caused by stasis below the site of obstruction in patients with venous thrombosis.[19-21] Hot spots may also be seen in the region of venous valves without disease (Fig. 11-11) or in calf veins that are without any venous disease or valves (Fig. 11-12). The reason for such entirely nonspecific hot spots in venograms has yet to be clarified.

EVALUATION OF SUPERIOR VENA CAVAL SYNDROME

Radionuclide venography may be used to evaluate superior vena caval obstructions. Obstruction of the superior vena cava, either by extrinsic compression or by thrombus, causes a characteristic clinical syndrome: cyanosis, swelling of the head, neck, and upper extremities, and development of superficial venous collateral vessels.[26] However, these signs may completely disappear when collateral vessels are well established.[27] Gradual obstruction may not cause obvious signs of superior vena caval syndrome, since collateral flows can be developed before there is a marked increase in pressure in the superior vena cava.

With the patient lying supine on an imaging table, the chest is aligned in the field of view of the camera and a 2-mCi dose of ^{99m}Tc-albumin particles is injected into an arm vein. Since the detection of a flow abnormality is the purpose of the study, any radiopharmaceutical may be used. If the patient needs a brain or liver scan, the respective imaging agent for those studies can be effectively used. Immediately after intravenous injection, dynamic flow images are obtained sequentially. If there is an obstruction of the superior vena cava, abnormal collateral flow through the superior intercostal vein, the hemiazygos vein, and even through the superior and inferior epigastric veins may be demonstrated on the superior vena cavograms (Fig. 11-13).

EVALUATION OF INFERIOR VENA CAVAL INTERRUPTIONS

Surgical interruption of venous flow, such as ligation of the vena cava or intravenous placement of a filter device or umbrella, is common practice in patients who develop recurrent pulmonary embolism despite satisfactory anticoagulation or who have bleeding complications, thus forcing discontinuation of anticoagulant therapy.[28] Unfortunately, recurrent embolization is not very uncommon after such surgical intervention.[29,30] Therefore, follow-up radionuclide vena cavography is a convenient technique for the evaluation of patency of intravenacaval filter devices or the status of collateral venous flow channels.

The patient is positioned under a scintillation camera lying supine on an imaging table. When a large-field-of-view camera is used, the venogram may be completed without moving the patient or imaging equipment because the camera field is large enough to cover the entire inferior caval vein in most cases.

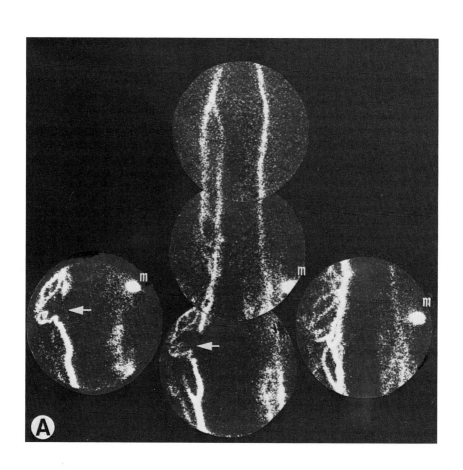

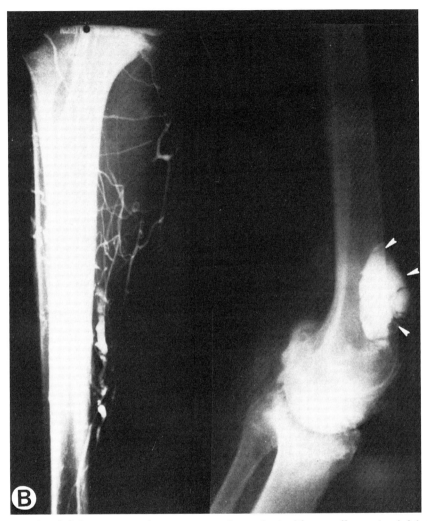

Figure 11-9. (A) Lower extremity venograms of a patient with a swollen and painful right lower leg show flow interruptions in the popliteal region (arrow) and distal femoral veins and extensive collateral channels. The deep veins of the left leg appear to be normal. A hot marker (m) was placed over the left knee. (B) A contrast venogram (left) of the right leg of the same patient shows collateral veins but without thrombosis of the deep veins. An arthrogram of the right knee (right) shows a large, cystic change (arrow head) in the suprapatellar bursa.

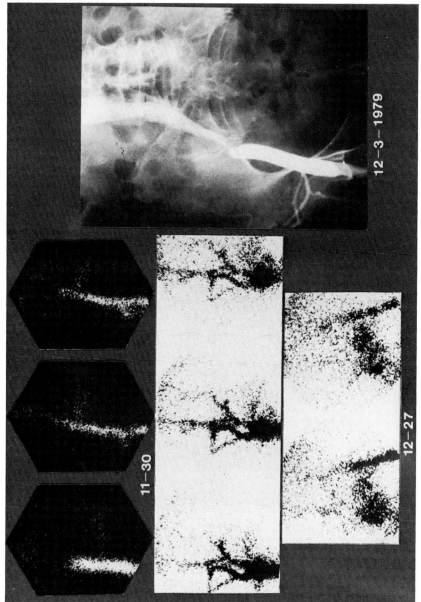

Figure 11-10. A follow-up evaluation of iliac vein patency after venous grafting. The first right iliac venogram (11-30) shows markedly reduced flow through the proximal iliac vein. The contrast venogram (12-3-1979) shows a severe stricture of the proximal end of the graft. A follow-up venogram (12-27) shows complete occlusion of the iliac vein and extensive collateral flow through the epigastric vein, the ascending lumbar vein, and into the left iliac vein through the collateral pelvic venous plexus.

226

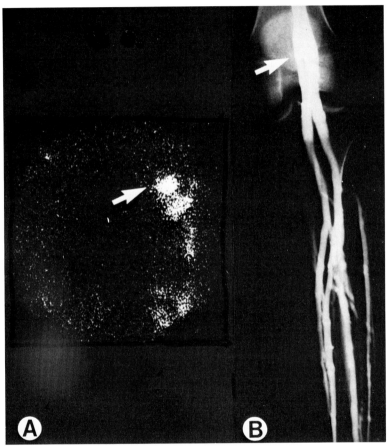

Figure 11-11. A venogram of the lower leg (A) showing "hot spots" (arrows). A contrast venogram obtained on the patient (B) showed that the hot spots corresponded to valves of the popliteal vein (arrows).

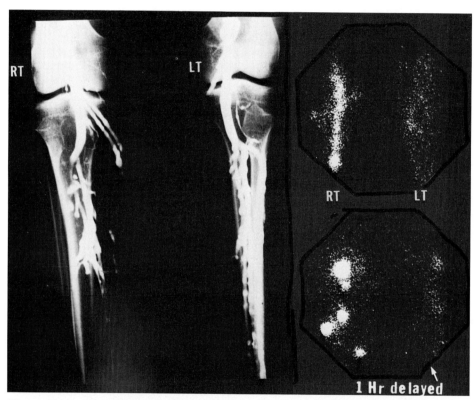

Figure 11-12. Essentially nonspecific "hot spots" in the calf veins. A venogram obtained on a patient with suspected thrombophlebitis shows abnormal stasis of radioactivity in the right calf (right, top). A 1-hour delayed scan (right, bottom) shows multiple hot spots. Contrast venograms of the patient (left), however, showed no abnormality in the calf veins. There were no varicosities corresponding to the hot spots.

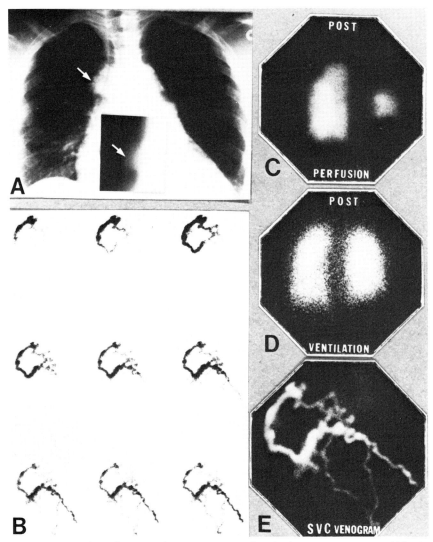

Figure 11-13. Radionuclide superior vena cavography. A chest roentgenogram (A) taken on a patient with suspected pulmonary embolism showed a questionable mass lesion in the right superior mediastinum (arrow). The possibility of obstruction of the superior vena cava was suggested but the patient showed no sign of the syndrome. Superior vena cavography was performed using ^{99m}Tc-MAA, because ventilation-perfusion lung scans were requested. The flow images (B) and a summed image (E) showed obstruction of the superior vena cava and extensive collateral veins. Subsequent perfusion and ventilation lung scans (C,D) showed a massive pulmonary embolism.

229

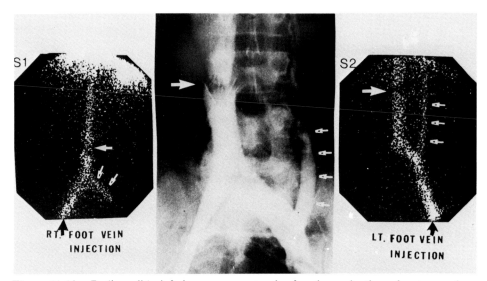

Figure 11-14. Radionuclide inferior vena cavography for the evaluation of patency of an inferior vena cava umbrella. (S1) A venogram with injection of ^{99m}Tc-MAA into the right leg shows a regurgitation into the left iliac vein (open arrows). (S2) When the injection was made into the left foot vein, collateral flow through the ascending lumbar vein was visualized (open arrows). The flow through the umbrella (large arrow) was not obstructed but it was causing significant stenosis of the caval vein.

A 1-to-2-mCi dose of ^{99m}Tc-albumin particles is injected into a foot vein and sequential inferior vena caval flow images are obtained. The use of a tourniquet in this technique is only for the intravenous injection. The injection may be made into one side of the leg, or both sides, but one side at a time (Fig. 11-14). However, the overall flow pattern and status of collateral channels can be better demonstrated when the injection is made into both legs simultaneously.

The entire collateral flow channels, from the leg to the chest, may be imaged in patients who have undergone inferior vena caval ligation by using a whole-body moving table technique (Fig. 11-15).

CONCLUSION

Simplicity and a reliability of over 90 percent, make radionuclide venography with ^{99m}Tc-albumin particles the best routine procedure for the evaluation of patients with suspected thromboembolic venous disease. Simultaneous visualization of the deep and superficial veins and imaging of the pelvic veins in lower extremity venography without additional injection are advantages with this technique. In particular, this is the only procedure in which perfusion lung images can be obtained immediately after a venogram without additional injections of radiopharmaceutical.

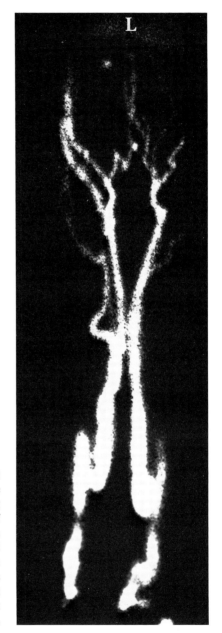

Figure 11.15. Radionuclide venogram in a patient who had had ligation of the inferior vena cava. The venogram was obtained using a whole-body scanning system after simultaneous bilateral injections of ^{99m}Tc-MAA into the dorsal foot veins. The flow is noted to be only through the superficial collateral channels, thus demonstrating complete obstruction of the inferior vena cava with satisfactory venous return through the extensive collateral veins. A faint image of the lung is seen at the top (L). The bottom of the image corresponds to the ankle of the patient.

REFERENCES

1. Dalen JE, Alpert JS: Natural history of pulmonary embolism. Prog Cardiovasc Dis 17:259–270, 1975

2. Sherry S: The problem of thromboembolic disease. Semin Nucl Med 7:205–211, 1977

3. Lambie JM, Mahaffy RG, Barber DC, et al: Diagnostic accuracy in venous thrombosis. Br Med J 2:142–143, 1970

4. Kakkar VV: Deep vein thrombosis. Circulation 51:8–19, 1975

5. Dos Santos JC: Phlebographic directe. Conception, technique, premiers resultants. J Int Chir 3:625–669, 1938

6. Rabinov K, Paulin S: Roentgen diagnosis of venous thrombosis in the leg. Arch Surg 104:134–144, 1972

7. Alberechtsson U, Olsson CG: Thrombotic side-effect of lower limb phlebography. Lancet 1:723–724, 1976

8. Kempi V, von Scheele C: Diagnosis of deep vein thrombosis with sodium pertechnetate. J Nucl Med 17:1096–1099, 1976

9. Vieras A, Barron EL, Parker GA: Evaluation of Tc-99m-sulfur-colloid uptake in experimental deep vein thrombosis (abstract). J Nucl Med 20:663, 1979

10. Stern HS, Zolle I, McAfee JG: Preparation of 99mTc-labeled serum albumin (human). Int J Appl Radiat 16:283–285, 1965

11. Gwyther MM, Field EO: Aggregated 99mTc-labeled albumin for lung scintiscanning. Int J Appl Radiat 17:485–489, 1966

12. Webber MM, Bennett LR, Cragin M, et al: Thrombophlebitis—demonstration by scintiscanning. Radiology 92:620–623, 1969

13. Rosenthal L, Greyson ND: Observations on the use of 99mTc-albumin macroaggregates for detection of thrombophlebitis. Radiology 94:413–416, 1970

14. Ryo UY, Colombetti LG, Polin SG, et al: Radionuclide venography: Significance of delayed washout, visualization of the saphenous system. J Nucl Med 17:590–595, 1976

15. Yao ST, Henkins RE, Conn J, et al: Combined isotope venography and lung scanning. Arch Surg 107:146–151, 1973

16. Henkins RE, Yao ST, Quinn JE, et al: Radionuclide venography (RNV) in lower extremity venous disease. J Nucl Med 15:171–175, 1974

17. Pollack EW, Webber MM, Victery W, et al: Radioisotope detection of venous thrombosis. Arch Surg 110:613–616, 1975

18. Van Kirk OC, Burry MT, Jansen AA, et al: A simplified approach to radionuclide venography. J Nucl Med 17:969–971, 1976

19. Hayt DB, Blatt CJ, Freeman LM: Radionuclide venography: Its place as a modality for the investigation of thromboembolic phenomena. Semin Nucl Med 7:263–281, 1977

20. Ryo UY, Qazi M, Strikantaswamy S, et al: Radionuclide venography: Correlation with contrast venography. J Nucl Med 18:11–17, 1977

21. Ennis JT, Elmes RJ: Radionuclide venography in the diagnosis of deep vein thrombosis. Radiology 125:441–449, 1977

22. Duffy GJ, D'Auria D, Brien TG, et al: New radioisotope test for detection of venous thrombosis in the legs. Br Med J 1:712–714, 1973

23. Webber MM, Victery W, Cragin MD: Demonstration of thrombophlebitis and endothelial damage by scintiscanning. Radiology 100:83–87, 1971

24. Driedger AA, Reid BD, Heagy FC: Lung and leg scanning with 99mTc-labeled albumin macroaggregated. Can Med Assoc J 11:403–405, 1974

25. Ryo UY, Lee JI, Pinsky SM: Radionuclide venography in the upper extremity. Clin Nucl Med 1:242–244, 1976

26. Sabiston DC Jr: Disease of the pleura, mediastinum and diaphragm, in Wintrobe MM, Thorn GW, Adams RD, et al (eds): Harrison's Principles of Internal Medicine, (ed 6). New York, McGraw-Hill, 1968, p 1348

27. Kumar B, Coleman RE, McKnight R: Asymptomatic superior vena cava obstruction. J Nucl Med 17:853–854, 1976

28. Davies GC, Salzman EW: The treatment of venous thrombosis and pulmonary embolism, in Joist JH, Sherman LA (eds): Venous and Arterial Thrombosis. New York, Grune & Stratton, 1978, pp 146–147

29. Mobbin-Uddin K, McLean R, Bolooki H, et al: Caval interruption for prevention of pulmonary embolism. Arch Surg 99:711–715, 1969

30. Piccone VA, Jr, Vidal E, Yarnoz M, et al: The late results of caval ligation. Surgery 68:980–998, 1970

31. Verma RC, Webber MM, Cragin MD: Correlation of 99mTc-MAA thrombosis scans to venograms (abstract). J Nucl Med 17:563, 1976

Joel Leland

12

Ultrasound and Computed Tomography of the Veins

The major venous structures of the body can be visualized by ultrasound[1-3] and by computed tomography (CT).[4,5] The inferior vena cava, the renal veins, and the ileo-femoral veins have received the most attention, since these vessels are most easily identified and lend themselves most readily to evaluation. Of these major venous channels, abnormalities of the inferior vena cava have been most frequently reported and these include thrombosis,[1,5,6] invasion by tumor with tumor thrombus (particularly in renal malignancies),[2,4,7-9] and congenital anomalies.[10-12]

All CT studies of these vascular structures should be performed following the administration of intravenous contrast material either as a bolus or by the drip infusion method. The rapid scanning time of the current generation of CT scanners permits the identification of the inferior vena cava in most patients without interference from motion artifacts. The faster scanning time allows rapid sequence dynamic scanning (4 to 5 scans in less than 1 minute) following a bolus injection of contrast.

With ultrasound, the superior portion of the inferior vena cava can be successfully demarcated in most patients with the distal portion occasionally being obscured by bowel gas. Using longitudinal and transverse scans, the position of the inferior vena cava (IVC) can be accurately defined as well as its relationship to surrounding structures. The IVC is best demonstrated in the longitudinal plane with the patient suspending respiration.[13] This serves to distend the vessel and allows the most satisfactory visualization. Suspension of breathing following a deep inspiration allows the liver to descend and act as an ultrasonic window for the structures posterior to it (Fig. 12-1).[3] A normal healthy patient can markedly distend the inferior vena cava with a Valsalva's maneuver (Fig. 12-2).[14] Persistent dilatation of the IVC, particularly in an older patient may be secondary to obstruction or to right-sided heart failure (Fig. 12-3). In the longitudinal projection, the distal and midportion of the IVC are horizontal in course, and the proximal portion is concave anteriorly[15] (Fig. 12-1). In the transverse

IMAGING OF THE PERIPHERAL VASCULAR SYSTEM Copyright © 1984 by Grune & Stratton.
ISBN 0-8089-1636-X

233

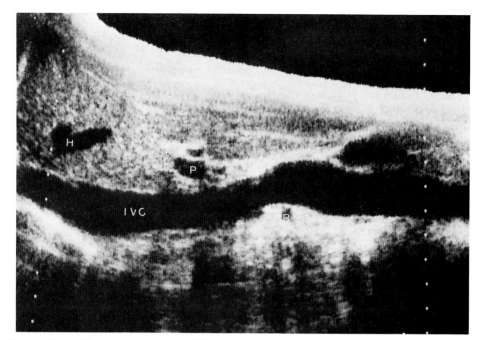

Figure 12-1. The inferior vena cava (IVC) from the diaphragm to a level below the umbilicus, near the origin of the IVC is demonstrated. I = IVC; R = right renal artery; H = hepatic veins; P = portal vein.

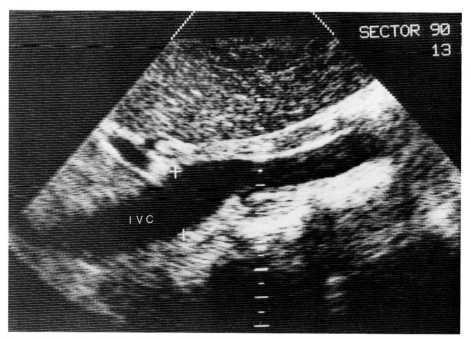

Figure 12-2. A well-distended proximal inferior vena cava following a Valsalva's maneuver.

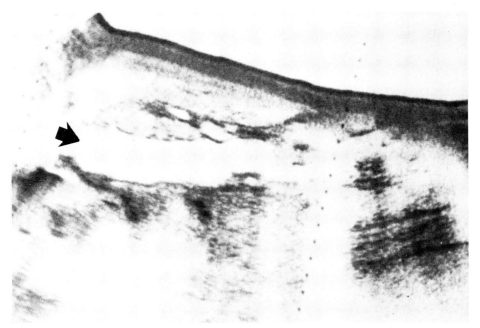

Figure 12-3. A persistently dilated inferior vena cava (arrow) in a patient with congestive heart failure.

projection, the IVC can be circular, triangular, or elliptical in shape (Fig. 12-4, A–C).

On CT scans, the femoral veins are seen at the level of the symphysis, medial to the femoral arteries, and anterior to the pectineus muscle (Fig. 12-5A). They continue cephalad, anterior to the acetabulum and femoral heads, and medial to the iliopsoas muscle (Fig. 12-5B). They then proceed as the iliac veins at the level of the upper sacrum, medial to the psoas muscle (Fig. 12-5C) and unite to form the IVC at the level of L-5 (Fig. 12-5D). From this point it ascends to the right of and anterior to the spine. In its caudal portion, it lies in close proximity to the spine but separates from it anteriorly as it moves cephalad to the right atrium. It is usually elliptical or oval in shape, and may get somewhat larger at the level of the renal veins. In its intrahepatic portion, it is separated from the portal vein by the caudate lobe (Fig. 12-5E).

Extension of renal carcinoma within the renal veins and IVC has been described.[2,4,5,8,9] The incidence of venous extension of renal cell carcinoma ranges from 9 to 33 percent.[15,16] The presence of renal tumor extension into the IVC adversely affects prognosis.[17] Since extension into the renal vein and IVC may alter the surgical approach,[18] it is important to determine the extent of the disease preoperatively. The demonstration of tumor thrombus is no longer an absolute contraindication to surgery.[19]

Diagnosis of venous thrombus by CT is made by using the indirect finding of massive enlargement of the venous diameter with an adjacent neoplasm (Fig. 12-6), or the direct finding of an intraluminal filling defect, which is best seen following the injection of intravenous contrast material. The thrombus is seen as an area of low density surrounded by blood containing iodine.[4,7,8]

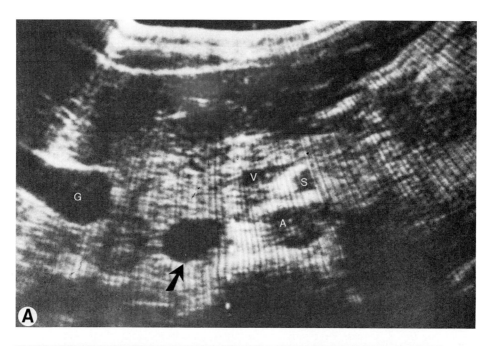

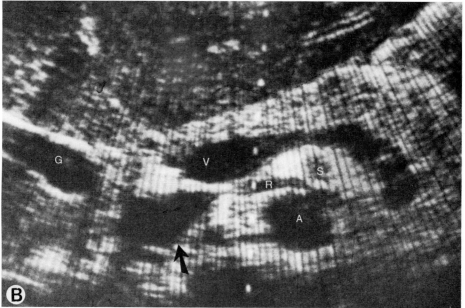

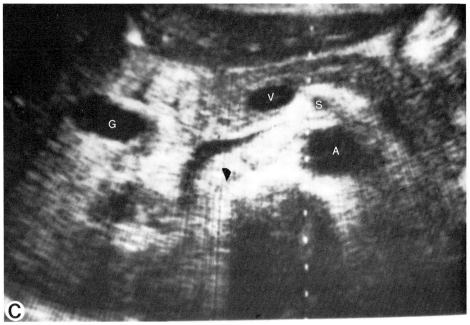

Figure 12-4. (A) Transverse scan of the inferior vena cava (IVC) (arrow) revealing a circular shape. A = aorta; S = superior mesenteric artery; V = superior mesenteric vein; G = gall bladder. (B) Triangular shape of the IVC (arrow) on a transverse scan (in same patient as in A). R = left renal vein. (C) Elliptical shape of the IVC (arrow).

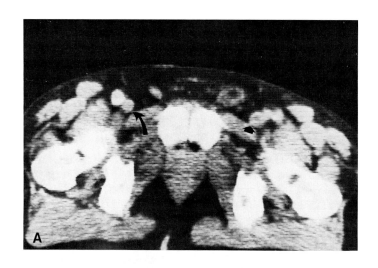

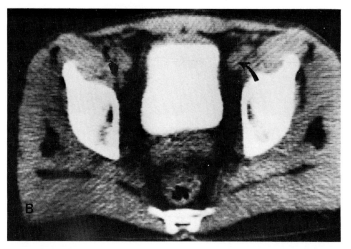

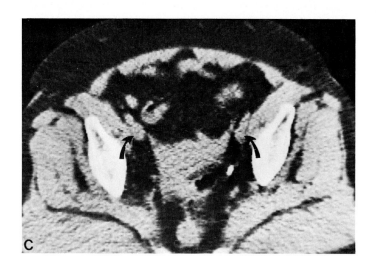

238

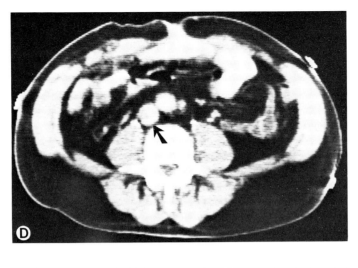

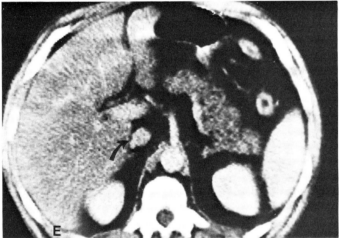

Figure 12-5. Computed tomographic scans of venous structures. (A) The femoral veins at the level of the symphysis (arrows). (B) The femoral veins at the level of the acetabulum (arrows). (C) The iliac veins at the level of the sacrum medial to the psoas muscle (arrows). (D) The IVC just proximal to its origin at L-5 (arrow). (E) The intrahepatic vena cava (arrow).

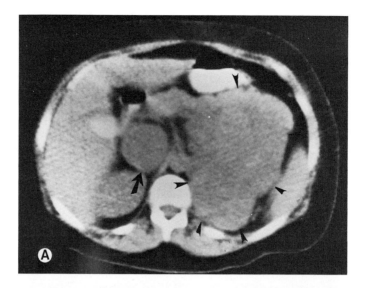

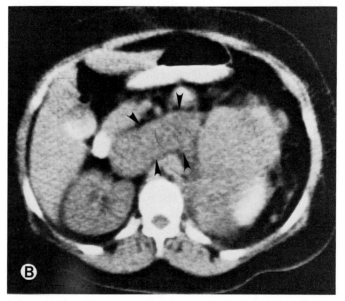

Figure 12-6. (A) A CT scan of the upper abdomen reveals a large mass (adrenal carcinoma) (arrowheads) and a dilated IVC (arrow). (B) A scan 2 cm caudal to that in A reveals an enlarged left renal vein (arrowheads). [Reprinted from Marks W, Korobkin M, Callen PE, et al: CT diagnosis of tumor thrombus of the renal vein and inferior vena cava. AJR 131:803–848, 1979. With Permission.]

Inferior vena caval and renal vein thrombosis can also be detected by ultrasound.[2,3,9] Once the diagnosis of a solid renal mass has been made, it is important to determine the extent of disease by evaluating the IVC and renal veins.[20] Tumor thrombus in the inferior vena cava appears as either a discrete echogenic mass or as

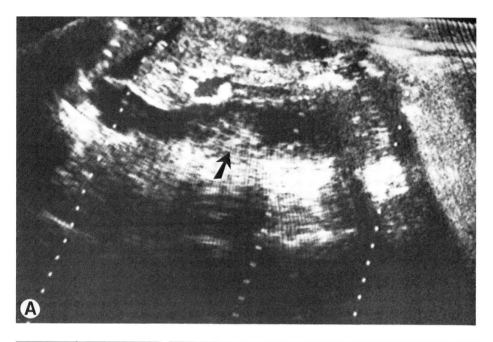

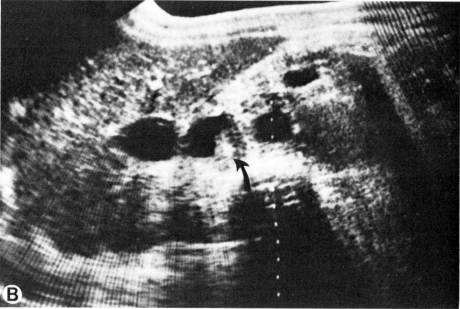

Figure 12-7. (A) A longitudinal scan 5 cm to right of midline reveals an echogenic mass (arrow) in the IVC. (B) A transverse scan reveals the mass (arrow) partially filling the IVC. Surgery confirmed metastatic hypernephroma.

diffuse echoes within the lumen[2,9] (Fig. 12-7). Ultrasound is also useful in demonstrating mass effects upon the cava of perivascular nodal masses in the prevertebral area, which may elevate the cava[3,21] (Fig. 12-8).

Thrombus in the ileofemoral veins (Fig. 12-9) and in the IVC other than of tumor origin has been described.[1,5,6] Although at the current time the diagnosis of venous thrombus is not a primary indication of computed tomography, its findings are characteristic, and it can be readily diagnosed by CT scan. The findings are similar to those for neoplastic invasion of the veins. They include enlargement of the thrombosed vein, a low-density lumen, and a sharply defined wall[5] (Fig. 12-10A,B).

Several studies have shown the time dependence of the attenuation values for clotted blood.[22–25] A recent thrombus may be as dense as contrast-enhanced blood and therefore not detectable in its early stages, but it will be later when its density increases.

Several anomalies of the inferior vena cava have been noted on CT scan. These include duplication of the inferior vena cava,[26–28] left-sided inferior vena cava,[27] and intrahepatic interruption with azygous continuation.[28,29]

In left-sided or transposition of the inferior vena cava, there is a single inferior vena cava to the left of the aorta; it crosses either anteriorly or posteriorly to the aorta at about the level of the renal arteries to reach the right atrium on the right side of the spine.[30] The ultrasonic appearance of this entity has been reported.[31]

In duplication of the inferior vena cava,[30,31] there is a normal IVC along the right side of the spine and a left-sided cava that ascends on the left of the aorta to join the right-sided cava at the level of the renal veins. Duplication of the IVC occurs with failure of regression of the left supracardinal vein. The incidence is 1 to 3 percent.[33] The duplicated IVC can be recognized by noting the separate drainage of the right and left renal veins into the right and left IVC and by observing the increased attenuation following intravenous contrast[27] (Fig. 12-11).

Azygous continuation of an anomalous inferior vena cava is found in 0.6 percent of children with congenital heart disease,[34] and it is also associated with polysplenia and asplenia syndromes.[35] It can also appear as an unexpected finding in patients without other anomalies. The plain film findings have been described and include a right paratracheal mass representing the azygous vein,[34] and the absence of the IVC shadow on the lateral chest film.[36]

The diagnosis on computed tomography can be suggested if a tubular structure is seen adjacent to the descending aorta, arching forward to join the superior vena cava at the level of the aortic arch, and forming a vascular ring around the trachea.[28,29] Enhancement of the dilated azygous vein following intravenous administration of contrast material will confirm the diagnosis (Fig. 12-12A–C).

Recognition of these anomalies is important to both the surgeon and the radiologist. Thoracotomies have been performed for mediastinal masses that proved to be enlarged azygous veins in patients with azygous continuation of the inferior vena cava.[37,38] Similar problems arise during nephrectomy or adrenalectomy in which venous hemorrhage occurs from accidental injury to a left inferior vena cava.[39] Another diagnostic pitfall is interpreting a double or left-sided vena cava as a lymph node mass. Enhancement with intravenous contrast could avoid this. Awareness by the radiologist of these anomalies could prevent unnecessary surgery or the morbidity that could result from injury to anomalous vessels during surgery.

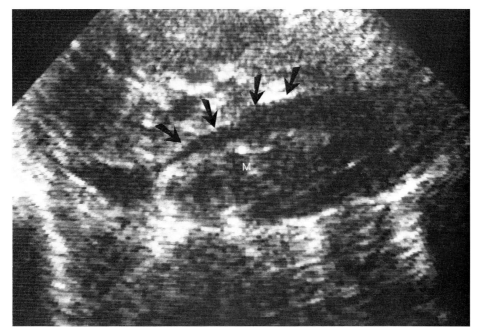

Figure 12-8. Longitudinal scan at the level of the IVC (arrows) reveals elevation of the IVC by a lymph node mass (**M**) posterior to it.

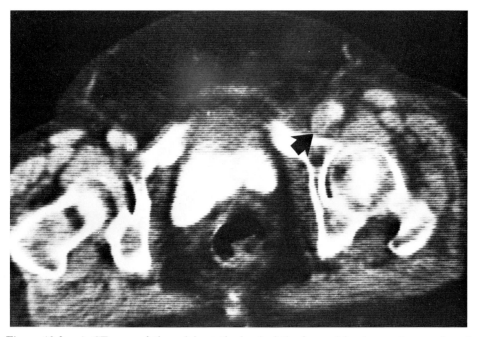

Figure 12-9. A CT scan of the pelvis at the level of the femoral heads reveals an enlarged left iliac vein with a low-density center representing thrombus surrounded by thin rim of contrast (arrow). R = right femoral vein.

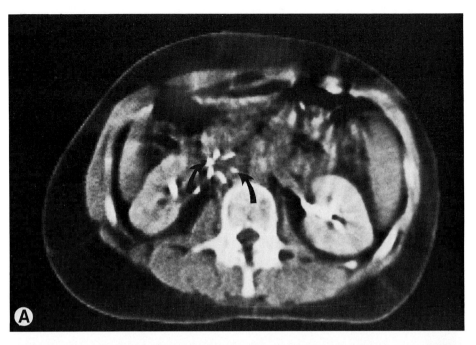

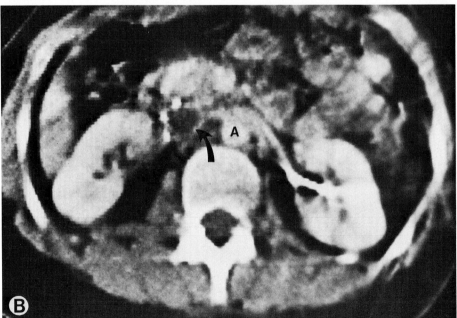

Figure 12-10. A patient with an umbrella and thrombus in the IVC (arrow). (A) A CT scan 9 cm below the umbilicus demonstrates umbrella in the IVC. (B) A scan 1.5 cm caudal to that in A reveals lower density center caused by thrombus when compared with aorta and a sharply defined lumen (arrow). A = aorta.

244

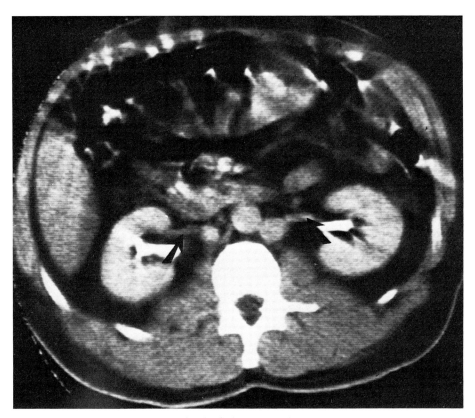

Figure 12-11. A CT scan at the level of the renal veins reveals right and left renal veins (arrows) emptying into the ipsilateral IVC, which is duplicated. [Reprinted from Breckenridge JW, Kinlaw WB: Azygous continuation of the inferior vena cava: CT appearance. J Comput Assist Tomogr 4:393–397, 1980. With permission.]

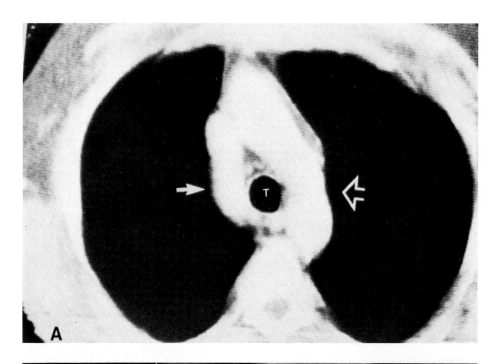

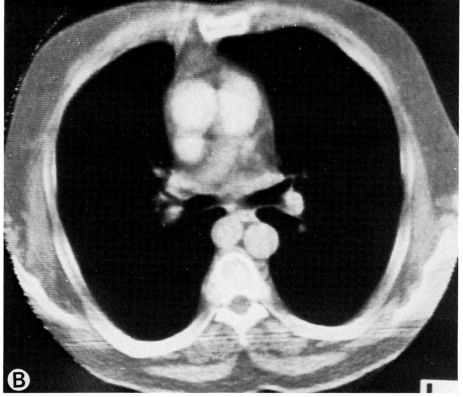

246

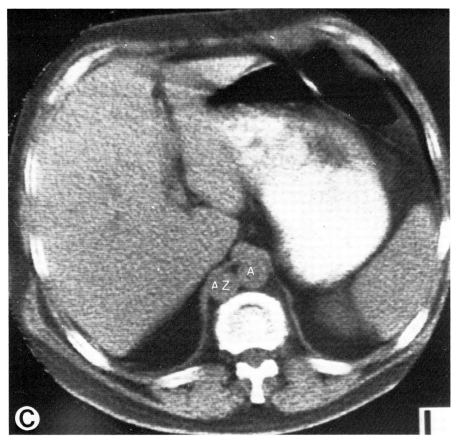

Figure 12-12. Azygous continuation of the IVC. (A) A CT scan of the chest shows dilated azygous arch (white arrow) paralleling aorta (open arrow). T = trachea. (B) A CT scan of the chest caudal to that in A shows dilated azygous vein (Az) to the right of the aorta (A). (C) A CT scan of the upper abdomen demonstrating retrocrural location of the azygous vein (Az). A = aorta. [Reprinted from Breckenridge JW, Kinlaw WB: Azygous continuation of the inferior vena cava: CT appearance. J Comput Assist Tomogr 4:393–397, 1980. With permission.]

REFERENCES

1. Sonnenfeld M, Finberg JH: Ultrasonic diagnosis of incomplete inferior vena cava thrombosis secondary to periphlebitis. Radiology 137:743–744, 1980

2. Goldstein HM, Green B, Weaver RM: Ultrasonic detection of renal tumor extension into the inferior vena cava. AJR 130:1083–1085, 1978

3. Gosink BB: The inferior vena cava: Mass effects. AJR 130:533–536, 1978

4. Marks WM, Korobkin M, Callen PW, et al: CT diagnosis of tumor thrombus of the renal vein and inferior vena cava. AJR 131:843–848, 1978

5. Zerhouni EA, Barth KH, Siegelman SS: Demonstration of venous thrombosis by computed tomography. AJR 134:753–758, 1980

6. Schmitz L, Jeffrey RB, Palubinskas AJ, et al: CT demonstration of septic thrombus of the inferior vena cava. J Comput Assist Tomogr 52:259–261, 1981

7. Dunnick NR, Doppman JL, Gelhoed GW: Intravenous extension of endocrine tumors. AJR 135:471–476, 1980

8. Steele JR, Sones PJ, Jeffries LT: The detection of inferior vena cava thrombosis with computed tomography. Radiology 128:385–386, 1978

9. Walzer A, Weiner SR, Koenigsberg M: The ultrasound appearance of tumor extension into the left renal veins and inferior vena cava. J Urol 123:945–946, 1980

10. Faer MJ, Lynch RD, Evans HO, et al: Inferior vena cava duplication: Demonstration by computed tomography. Radiology 130:707–709, 1975

11. Royal SA, Calla PW: CT evaluation of anomalies of the inferior vena cava and left renal vein. AJR 112:759–763, 1979

12. Garris JB, Kangarloo H, Sample WF: Ultrasonic diagnosis of intrahepatic interruption of the inferior vena cava with azygous (hemiazygous) continuation. Radiology 134:179–183, 1980

13. Grant E, Randero F, Servinc E: Normal inferior vena cava: Caliber changes observed by dynamic ultrasound. AJR 135:335–338, 1980

14. Filly RA, Goldberg BB: Normal vessels, in Goldberg BB (ed): Abdominal Gray Scale Ultrasonography. New York, John Wiley & Sons, 1977, pp 26–31

15. Robsan CJ, Church BRN, Anderson W: The results of radical nephrectomy for renal cell carcinoma. J Urol 101:297–301, 1969

16. McCoy RM, Klatte EL, Rhamy RK: Use of inferior vena cavography in the evaluation of renal neoplasms. J Urol 102:556–559, 1969

17. Ney C: Thrombosis of inferior vena cava associated with malignant renal tumors. J Urol 55:583–590, 1946

18. McCullough DL, Talner LB: Inferior vena caval extension of renal carcinoma: A lost cause? AJR 131:819–826, 1979

19. Skinner DG, Pfister RF, Colvin N: Extension of renal cell carcinoma into the vena cava: The rationale for aggressive surgical management. J Urol 107:711–716, 1972

20. Green B, Goldstein HM, Weaver RM: Abdominal pansonography in the evaluation of renal cancer. Radiology 132:421–424, 1979

21. Kurtz AF, Rubin C, Goldberg BB: Ultrasound diagnosis of masses elevating the inferior vena cava. AJR 132:401–410, 1979

22. Dolinskas CA, Bulgniuk LT, Zimmerman RA, et al: Computed tomography of intracerebral hematoma: Transmission CT observations on hematoma resolution. AJR 129:581–688, 1970

23. Korobkin M, Moss AA, Calla PW, et al: Computed tomography of subcapsular splenic hematome resolutions. Radiology 129:441–445, 1978

24. Bergstron M, Ericson K, Levander B, et al: Variation with time of the attenuation values of intracranial hematomas. J Comput Assist Tomogr 1:57–63, 1977

25. Messina AV, Chernik ML: Computed tomography: The "resolving" intracranial hemorrhage. Radiology 118:609–613, 1976

26. Faer MJ, Lynch RD, Evans IJA, et al: Inferior vena cava duplication: Demonstration by computed tomography. Radiology 130:707–709, 1979

27. Royal SA, Callen PW: CT evaluation of anomalies of the inferior vena cava and left renal veins. AJR 132:759–763, 1979

28. Breckenridge JW, Kinlaw WB: Azygous continuation of inferior vena cava: CT appearance. J Comput Assist Tomogr 4:393–397, 1980

29. Hill II RJ, Wesby G, Massan RE, et al: Computed tomographic demonstration of anomalous inferior vena cava with azygous continuation. J Comput Assist Tomogr 4:398–402, 1980

30. Brener BJ, Darling KC, Frederick PL, et al: Major venous anomalies complicating abdominal aorta surgery. Arch Surg 108:159–165, 1979

31. Tagin JS, Henderson MR, Smith AP: Sonographic demonstration of left sided inferior vena cava with hemiazygous continuation. AJR 134:1057–1059, 1980

32. Chuang VP, Mera CE, Hoskins PA: Congenital anomalies of the IVC; Review of the embryogenesis and presentation of a simplified classification. Br J Radiol 47:206–213, 1979

33. Hirsch DM, Cha KF: Bilateral inferior vena cava. JAMA 185:729–730, 1963

34. Berdan WE, Baker DH: Plain film findings in azygous continuation of the inferior vena cara. AJR 104:452–457, 1968

35. Vaughan TJ, Hawkins IF, Elliot LP: Diagnosis of polysplenia syndrome. Radiology 101:511–518, 1971

36. Heller RM, Dorst JP, James AW, et al: A useful sign in the recognition of azygous continuation of the inferior vena cava. Radiology 101:519–522, 1971

37. Floyd DG, Nelson WP: Developmental interruption of the inferior vena cava with azygous and hemiazygous substitution. Radiology 119:55–57, 1976

38. Petersen RW: Infrahepatic interruption of the inferior vena cava with azygous continuation: Persistent right cardinal vein. Radiology 84:304–307, 1965

39. Sethuk PJ, Mysosekan UR, Pstil TL: Double inferior vena cava. Indian J Med Sci 25:334–339, 1971

Siddalingappa Srikantaswamy

13
Contrast Venography

FEMORAL VEIN

The technique of femoral vein puncture at the groin is similar to that for puncture of the femoral artery except that the puncture site is 1 cm medial to the artery. A 16- or 18-gauge Teflon sheathed needle is inserted while the artery is retracted laterally. Simultaneous transfixation of the artery and vein should be avoided. If there is accidental transfixation of both the artery and vein, arterial bleeding must be controlled before another attempt is made to puncture the vein. After the vein is punctured, aspiration through the sheath with a syringe will result in venous return.

LOWER EXTREMITY VEINS

The veins of the lower extremities are opacified by contrast material through 19- or 21-gauge needles inserted into dorsal veins of the feet. The stability of the inserted needle is checked by a moderately forceful injection of normal saline. Diluted contrast medium (50 ml of contrast plus 25 ml of normal saline) is injected through the needle. Application of tight tourniquets, one above each ankle and one above each knee, before injection will facilitate better opacification of the deeper veins of the calf. After the entire amount of contrast medium has been injected, two successive films of the calf are obtained. Then one film of the thigh and one film of the pelvis are obtained after the tourniquets are removed. To avoid stasis of the contrast medium in the veins, 200 ml of normal saline is flushed into the veins immediately. During filming, slight flexion of the knee will eliminate spurious obstructions caused by surrounding normal structures (Fig. 13-1). In some instances an additional study in the lateral projection may also be indicated.

IMAGING OF THE PERIPHERAL VASCULAR SYSTEM Copyright © 1984 by Grune & Stratton.
ISBN   0-8089-1636-X   All rights of reproduction in any form reserved.

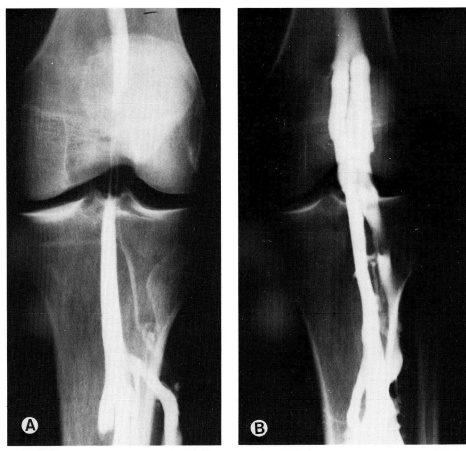

Figure 13-1. (A) Narrowing of the popliteal vein at the popliteal fossa. (B) The same patient after flexion of the knee.

A delayed film may better demonstrate venous thrombi. In cases of extensive thrombosis of the veins, when there are no injectable veins in the foot, any suitable superficial vein in the calf or thigh can be used. This will yield satisfactory diagnostic information. In an individual with swelling of the entire lower extremity, it is advisable to obtain a conventional lower extremity venogram by injecting a pedal vein, if possible. This will avoid unsuccessful puncture of a thrombosed femoral vein.

Lower extremity venograms can also be obtained while the patient is in a semierect or erect position. When such positions are used, there may be undue stasis of contrast in the veins because of gravity. In such situations, immediate flushing with normal saline is suggested. Descending venography can be undertaken to demonstrate the locations of incompetent veins, and to evaluate postsurgical results[1] (Fig. 13-2).

UPPER EXTREMITY VEINS

The technique for contrast venography of the upper extremities is essentially similar to that of lower extremity venography. A vein in the dorsum of the hand or a vein in the antecubital fossa is used for injection of the contrast medium. Tourniquets, one above each wrist and one above each antecubital fossa will facilitate better opacification of the deep veins.

INFERIOR VENACAVOGRAPHY

Both femoral veins are punctured at the groin and a total of 48 ml of contrast medium is injected through a "Y" connector over 4 seconds. During injection, filming is done at one film per second for 8 seconds over the abdomen to include the pelvis. When the studies are being done for thromboembolic abnormalities, both iliac veins should be visualized along with the inferior vena cava. Such an approach will avoid overlooking venacaval developmental abnormalities[2,3] (Fig. 13-3).

THE SUPERIOR VENA CAVA AND ITS TRIBUTARIES

Essentially, the technique for superior venacavography is similar to that for inferior venacavography. Both antecubital veins in their fossa are used for injection of the contrast medium. Preferably, 18-gauge teflon sleeves are introduced. A total of 48 ml of contrast medium over 4 seconds is injected through a "Y" connector. If the superior vena cava needs to be opacified further, a total of 60 ml of contrast is injected over 5 seconds.

VENOUS ANATOMY OF THE LOWER EXTREMITIES

The great saphenous vein[4] which begins medially in the foot, terminates at the femoral vein a little below the inguinal ligament. The short saphenous vein, which begins laterally, ends in the popliteal fossa.

The deep veins of the calf accompany the arteries. The popliteal vein becomes the femoral vein at the adductor canal, which in turn ends at the inguinal ligament to course as the external iliac vein.

VENOUS ANATOMY OF THE UPPER EXTREMITIES

The superficial veins[4] of the upper extremities are the cephalic vein, starting laterally in the hand, the basilic vein, starting medially, and the median vein, which drains the superficial palmar venous plexus. The deep veins are the radial and ulnar veins, which in turn course as the brachial vein into the axillary vein and then on to the subclavian vein, which in turn merges into the innominate vein.

Venous thrombosis is usually caused by stasis or hyperviscosity or by structural changes in the wall of the vessel.[5] When there is thrombus in a vein, embolization may occur during the first week as a result of loose thrombus. After a few weeks, the thrombus becomes adherent and retracts to be followed by recanalization. Organization and recanalization[6–9] of a thrombus are independent reparative processes. Complete recanalization of a thrombus occurs between the vessel wall and the clot (Figs. 13-4, 13-5).

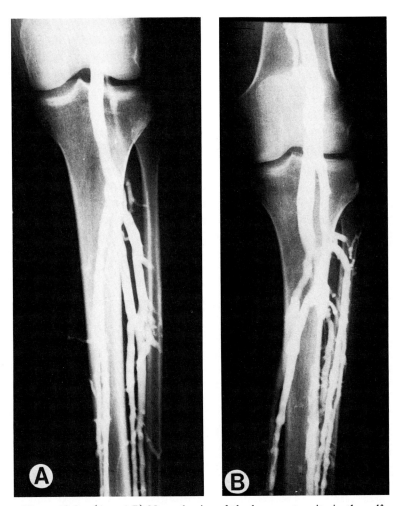

Figure 13-2. (A and B) Normal veins of the lower extremity in the calf.

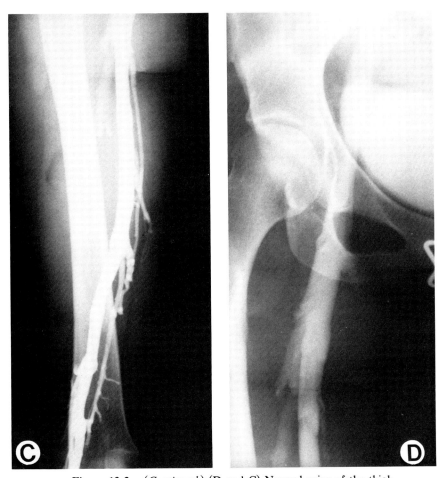

Figure 13-2. (*Continued.*) (D and C) Normal veins of the thigh.

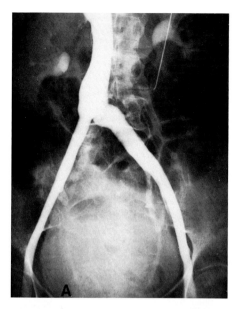

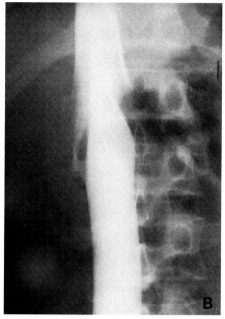

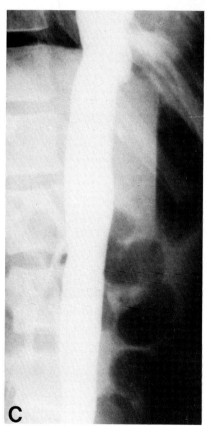

Figure 13-3. (A) Normal iliac veins. (B) Anteroposterior and (C) lateral views of the inferior vena cava.

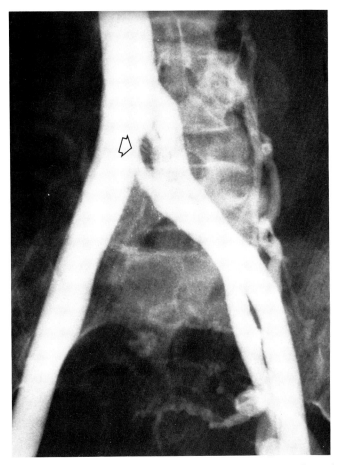

Figure 13.4 Linear and oval (arrow) filling defects in the left common iliac vein as a result of organization and recanalization of a thrombus.

In the lower extremities, the usual involvement is that of the deep veins of the calf. Thrombosis of the veins of the foot is not uncommon and can occur independently without associated calf vein involvement. In certain instances they may be the only source of pulmonary emboli.[10] Silent iliofemoral venous thrombosis may be a frequent occurrence in women using oral contraceptives,[11] in flaccid paraplegic individuals,[12] or prosthetic hip surgery. Iliocaval thrombosis causes a higher incidence of pulmonary embolism when compared with thrombosis of the calf veins.[13] Phlegmasia cerulea dolens,[14,15,16] a severe form of venous thrombosis, presents itself as a painful, purplish-blue, cold extremity with absent pulses. If it is not treated immediately, gangrene may be the outcome. Postvenography thrombosis can occur as a result of large doses of undiluted contrast medium in normal veins,[17] and venous gangrene[18] can develop in individuals with associated venous thrombosis (Figs. 13-6–13-10).

Collapsible normal veins are easily subjected to pseudoobstructions from adjacent muscles or osseous structures. Unopacified blood from a tributary draining into a major vein may lead the interpreter astray if he or she is unaware of such artifacts.

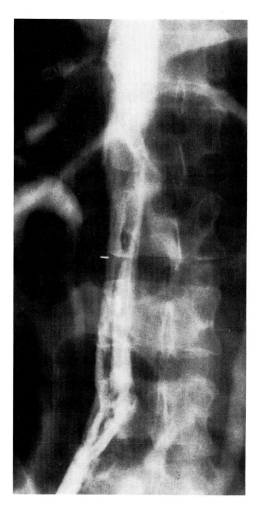

Figure 13-5. Linear filling defects in the inferior vena cava as a result of organization and recanalization of a thrombus.

Thrombosis of the inferior vena cava in its lower third is usually caused by propagation of extremity venous thrombosis. In its middle portions, renal pathologic entities, and adrenal or pancreatic neoplasms contribute to the etiology. The upper third of the vena cava can be extrinsically compressed by hepatic masses and lymph nodal processes. Occasionally, retroperitoneal fibrosis, tumors of the cava, trauma, or congenital diaphragms can cause occlusion at various levels (Figs. 13-11, 13-12).

Subclavian Vein Thrombosis

Because of its location, the subclavian vein is exposed to extrinsic pressure from adjacent normal structures of the thoracic outlet. It can also be encased by pulmonary neoplasms. Intrinsically, unusual effort or prolonged pressure on the vein as a result of eccentric positioning of the extremity[19] can cause venous thrombosis (Fig. 13-13).

Radical mastectomy deserves special mention, since the subclavian vein and its branches could be encased in recurrent tumor or entrapped in scar tissue or thrombosed, either because of thrombophelbitis or radiation.[20,21]

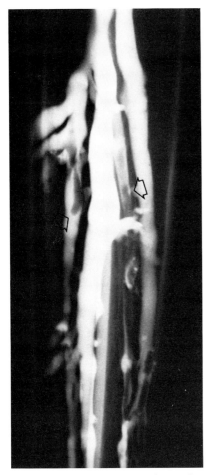 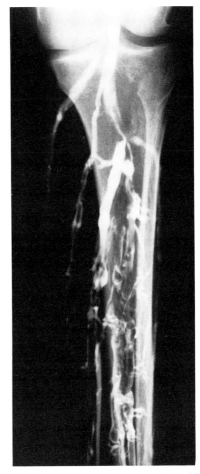

Figure 13-6. Loose thrombi (arrows) in the deep veins of the calf.

Figure 13-7. Extensive acute thrombi of the deep veins of the calf.

Hypertrophied valves[22] (Fig. 13-14) and diaphragms[23] are rare causes of obstruction of the vein.

Thrombosis of the Superior Vena Cava

A frequent cause of superior venacaval thrombosis is usually primary pulmonary malignancies, particularly the anaplastic variety.[24] Other benign and malignant mediastinal processes have the potential to cause superior venacaval thrombosis, including granulomatous diseases, ventriculoatrial shunt catheters,[25] fibrosing mediastinitis,[26] aortic aneurysms, transvenous cardiac pacemakers,[27,28] and hyperalimentation lines.

Miscellaneous causes of venous occlusion include tumoral emboli (Figs. 13-15–13-21) lymphosarcoma,[29] malignant tumors,[30] vessel wall tumors,[31] and congenital bands.[32]

Traumatic lesions of the veins include lacerations, hematomas, and thrombosis.[33]

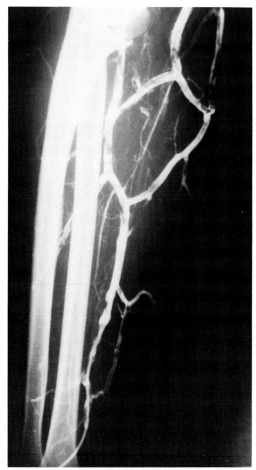

Figure 13-8. Nonfilling of the deep veins and loose thrombi in the superficial veins of the forearm.

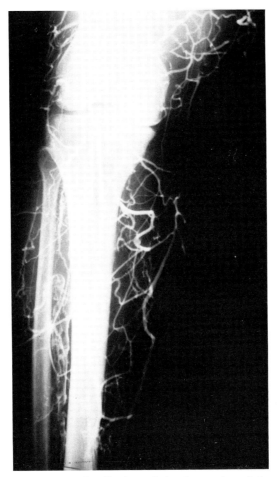

Figure 13-9. Nonvisualization of the deep veins of the calf with extensive collateral circulation through the superficial veins as a result of complete acute thrombosis of the deep veins.

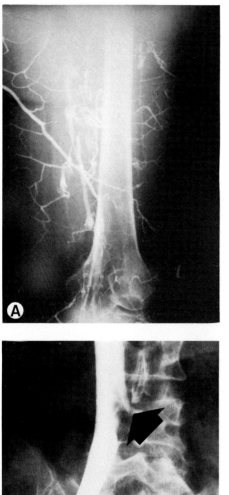

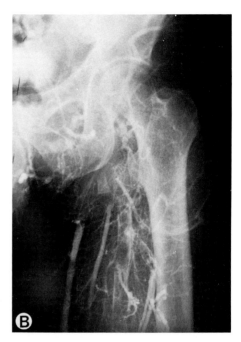

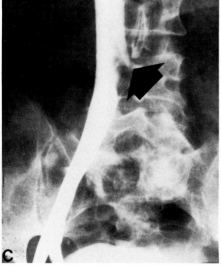

Figure 13-10. Complete thrombosis of the deep veins of the left lower extremity (A,B) with extension of the thrombus to the bifurcation of the vena cava (arrow) (C).

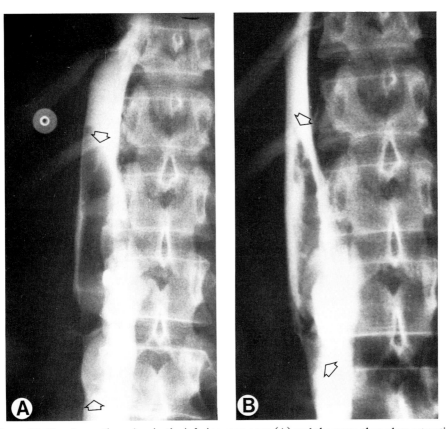

Figure 13-11. Loose thrombus in the inferior vena cava (A) and the same thrombus retracting (B) 3 months later.

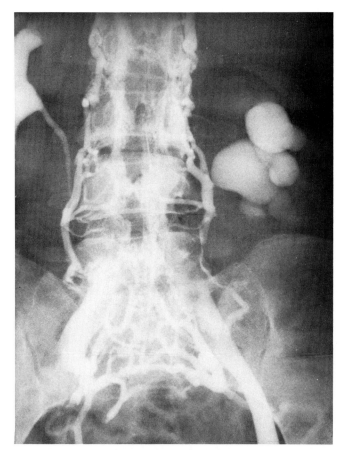

Figure 13-12. Nonvisualization of the inferior vena cava and collateral circulation through the vertebral plexus. The findings were caused by metastatic entrapment by a breast carcinoma. Also note the ureteral entrapment, causing hydronephrosis.

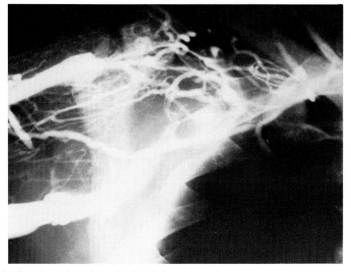

Figure 13-13. Complete thrombosis of the subclavian vein caused by excessive effort.

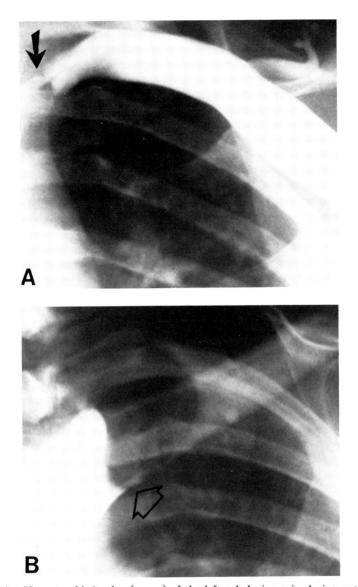

Figure 13-14. Hypertrophied valve (arrow) of the left subclavian vein during antegrade (A) and retrograde (B) injections. There is obvious flow obstruction during both phases. This individual had dependent edema that was relieved by elevation of that arm.

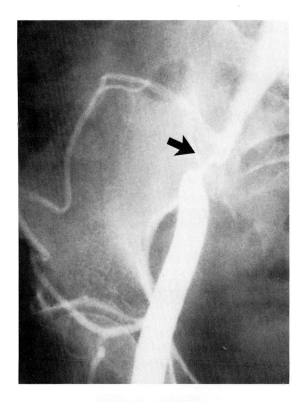

Figure 13-15. Marked stenosis (arrow) of the right iliac vein as a result of encasement by an ovarian malignancy.

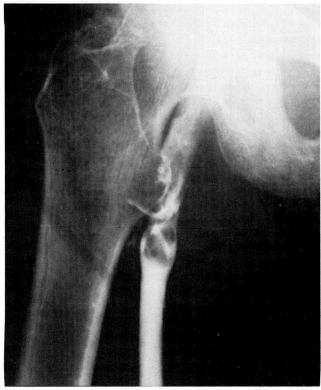

Figure 13-16. An expanding filling defect in the superior femoral vein as a result of metastatic breast carcinoma.

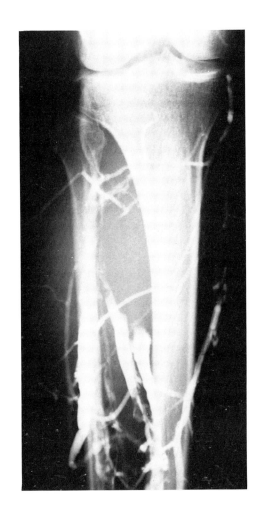

Figure 13-17. Abrupt terminations and displacement of the deep veins as a result of a traumatic hematoma.

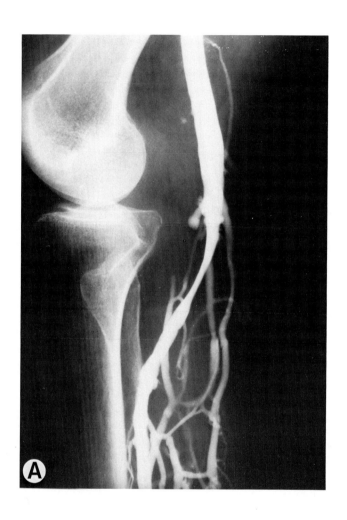

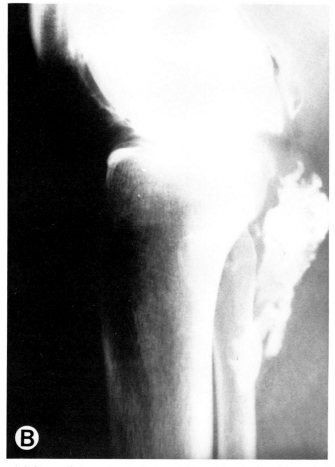

Figure 13-18. (A) (Lateral) Posterior deviation of the popliteal vein with extrinsic compression. (B) Knee arthrogram reveals a ruptured Baker's cyst.

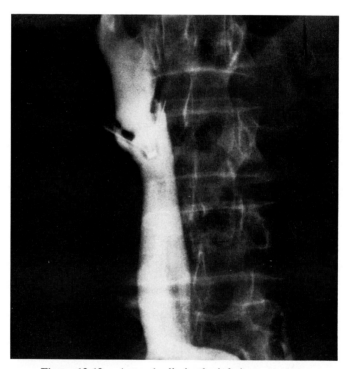

Figure 13-19. An umbrella in the inferior vena cava.

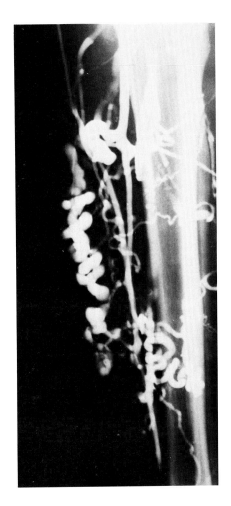

Figure 13-20. Incompetent communicating veins of the calf.

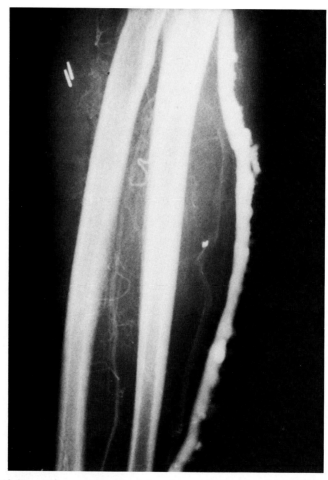

Figure 13-21. Atheromatous ulcers in a forearm vein caused by a dialysis shunt.

REFERENCES

1. Herman RJ, Yao J, Nieman H, et al: Descending venography. Radiology 137:63–69, 1980

2. Pillari G, Wind ES, Wiener SL, et al: Left inferior vena cava. AJR 130:366–367, 1978

3. Floyd GD, Nelson WP: Developmental interruption of the inferior vena cava with azygos and hemiazygos substitution. Radiology 119:55–57, 1976

4. Warwick R, Williams PL (eds): Gray's Anatomy. Philadelphia, W.B. Saunders, 1973

5. Virchow, cited by Fontaine R: John Homan's memorial lecture: Remarks concerning venous thrombosis and its sequelae. Surgery 41:6–25, 1957

6. Robbins SL: Pathologic Basis of Disease. Philadelphia, W.B. Saunders, 1975

7. Dible JH: Organization and canalization in arterial thrombosis. J Pathol Bacteriol 75:1–6, 1958

8. Filshie I, Scott GBD: The organization of experimental venous thrombi. J Pathol Bacteriol 76:71–77, 1958

9. Cox JST: Maturation and canalization of thrombi. Surg Gynecol Obstet 116:593–599, 1963

10. Thomas ML, O'Dwyer JA: A phlebographic study of the incidence and significance of venous thrombosis in the foot. AJR 135:751–752, 1978

11. Brodelius A, Lorenc P, Nylander G: Localization of acute deep venous thrombosis in women taking contraceptives. Radiology 101:297–300, 1971

12. Pors E, Conrad CA, Massel TB: Venous occlusion of lower extremities in paraplegic patients. Surg Gynecol Obstet 99:451, 454, 1954

13. Gibbs NM: Venous thrombosis of the lower extremity with particular reference to bed rest. Br J Surg 45:209–236, 1957

14. Lipchik EO, Altman DP: Phlegmasia cerulea dolens. Radiology 133:81–82, 1979

15. Brockman SK, Vasco JSK: Observation on the pathophysiology and treatment of phlegmasia cerulea alba dolens. Am J Surg 109:485–490, 1965

16. Stallworth JM, Eisenstein J: Phlegmasia cerulea dolens, a 10 year review. Ann Surg 161:802–809, 1965

17. Bettman MA, Salzman EW, Rosenthal D, et al: Reduction of venous thrombosis complicating phlebography. AJR 134:1169–1172, 1980

18. Thomas ML: Gangrene following peripheral phlebography. Br J Radiol 43:528–530, 1970

19. Adams JT, McEvoy RK, Deweese JA: Primary deep venous thrombosis of the upper extremity. Arch Surg 91:29–42, 1965

20. Gallagher PG, Algird JR: Post radical mastectomy edema of the arm. Angiography 17:377–387, 1966

21. Russo PE, Parker JM, Mathews HH, et al: Changes of the axillary vein after radical mastectomy. South Med J 47:430–436, 1954

22. Wilder JR, Habermann ET, Nach RL: Subclavian vein obstruction secondary to hypertrophy of the valve. Surgery 55:214–219, 1964

23. Cucil CT, Bottino CG, Ciampa V, et al: Venous obstruction of the upper extremity caused by a malformed valve of the subclavian vein. Circulation 27:275–278, 1963

24. Szur L, Bromley LL; Obstruction of the superior vena cava in carcinoma of the bronchus. Br Med J 2:1273–1276, 1956

25. Cha EM, Khoury G, Waly FAK: Collateral circulation in superior venacaval obstruction following ventriculoatrial shunt catherization. Radiology 102:605–611, 1972

26. Hansen KF: Idiopathic fibrosis of the mediastinum as a cause of superior venacaval syndrome. Radiology 85:433–438, 1965

27. Wertheimer M, Hughes RK, Castle H: Superior vena cava syndrome. JAMA 224:1172–1173, 1973

28. Chamorro H, Rao G, Wholey M: Superior vena cava syndrome, a complication of transvenous pacemaker implantation. Radiology 126:377–378, 1978

29. Ferris E: Venography of inferior vena cava and its branches. Baltimore, Williams & Wilkins, 1969

30. Lagergren C, Lindbom A, Soderberg G: Angiographic demonstration of a tumor thrombus in the popliteal vein. Acta Radiol (Diag) 52:401–405, 1959

31. Light HG, Peskin GW: Primary tumors of the venous system. Cancer 13:818–824, 1960

32. Negus D, Fletcher EWL: Compression and band formation at the mouth of the left common iliac vein. Br J Surg 55:369–374, 1968

33. Gerlock AJ, Muhletaler CA: Venography of peripheral venous injuries. Radiology 133:77–80, 1979

Jonathan E. Hasson
Steven A. Gould
Gerald S. Moss

14

Blood Flow Laboratory Evaluation of the Carotid Arteries

Stroke is a major cause of death and disability in the United States. It has been estimated that 12,500 strokes per one million persons occur each year, and that these are associated with a 30-day mortality of 40 percent.[1] Approximately 30 to 50 percent of patients with cerebral infarction have had a previous transient ischemic attack (TIA).[2] In those patients with untreated TIAs, approximately one third will progress to stroke.[3] Several studies have demonstrated a 40-percent incidence of isolated, surgically accessible lesions of the extracranial carotid system in patients with TIAs or stroke[4,5] The early detection of correctible carotid disease is therefore important if morbidity and mortality from stroke are to be decreased.

Arteriography remains the most definitive technique for the diagnosis of significant extracranial occlusive disease of the carotid artery system. The time, expense, and small though significant risk associated with contrast arteriography preclude its use as a routine technique for screening or follow-up of this disease.[5,6] Multiple noninvasive methods for the diagnosis of carotid occlusive disease have therefore been developed and have taken on much importance in recent years. These techniques allow several problems that arise in the management of carotid disease to be addressed.

In patients with asymptomatic bruits, the techniques can be used to determine if hemodynamically significant disease is present. In the presence of vague or non-hemispheric symptoms, it can be determined if the bruit is associated with extracranial carotid disease. In a preoperative patient in whom significant blood loss or hypotension is expected, the techniques can be used to determine if a significant stenotic lesion is present that might increase the risk of stroke.

The techniques can also be used for preoperative diagnosis in patients with tias or stroke, postoperative diagnosis and follow-up, and for following the natural history of asymptomatic bruits and stenoses.

IMAGING OF THE PERIPHERAL VASCULAR SYSTEM Copyright © 1984 by Grune & Stratton.
ISBN 0-8089-1636-X

There are multiple techniques for noninvasive diagnosis of extracranial carotid occlusive disease that will be discussed. These include periorbital Doppler examination, periorbital PPG examination, carotid phonoangiography, oculoplethysmography (pulse arrival time and Gee pneumoplethysmography), and spectral bruit analysis.

It should be stated at the outset that these techniques are not especially valuable in the diagnosis of plaque disease of the carotid system; they are primarily directed toward the detection of significant stenosis causing hemodynamic changes. A hemodynamically significant lesion; i.e., one that will produce a significant pressure drop and alteration of flow characteristics, is one that reduces the cross-sectional area of the internal carotid by 75 percent (diameter reduction of 50 percent). Lesions smaller than these are not thought to affect flow characteristics, although they may be the source of emboli.

PERIORBITAL DOPPLER EXAMINATION

In the presence of significant internal carotid stenosis or occlusion, those areas supplied by the normal distribution of this vessel will often receive collateral flow from other extracranial or intracranial vessels. It is the detection of this presence of collateral flow that is the basis of the periorbital Doppler technique.[7]

The internal carotid artery gives rise to only one extracranial branch—the ophthalmic artery. This vessel gives off three branches; the frontal, the supraorbital, and the nasal arteries. The superficial temporal and facial arteries (branches of the external carotid) form anastomotic networks with the ophthalmic artery branches (facial–nasal and superficial temporal–supraorbital/frontal) (Fig. 14-1).

There is another significant communication between the internal carotid arteries of both sides of the neck via the anterior communicating artery of the circle of Willis. There are then three major collateral systems that can be studied: the ipsilateral extracranial-intracranial (EC-IC) system (superficial temporal–frontal, supraorbital); the ipsilateral EC-IC system (facial–nasal); and the contralateral IC-IC system (anterior cerebral–anterior communicating (Willis)–anterior cerebral).

Normally, flow in the branches of the ophthalmic artery is directed outward from the orbit (Fig. 14-1). With the use of directional Doppler ultrasound (which can determine the direction of flow), the branches of the ophthalmic artery are examined for reversal of flow, i.e., flow directed into the orbit. If reversed flow is found, this implies that collateral flow is being provided from the ipsilateral external carotid. The implication of this finding is the presence of a stenosis in the diameter of the internal carotid on that side that is greater than 50 percent (Fig. 14-2).

In the absence of spontaneous flow reversal in the ophthalmic artery branches, the flow is then examined in response to compression of the branches of the external carotid. The superficial temporal artery is compressed first. In a normal carotid system, compression of the superficial temporal artery will cause augmentation or no change of flow in the supraorbital or frontal artery. A decrease or loss of the Doppler signal on compression is considered to demonstrate the presence of collateral flow from the external carotid, and suggests a significant internal carotid stenosis or occlusion.

Finally, collaterals from the contralateral internal carotid may be sought by compressing the contralateral common carotid low in the neck. If the supraorbital or

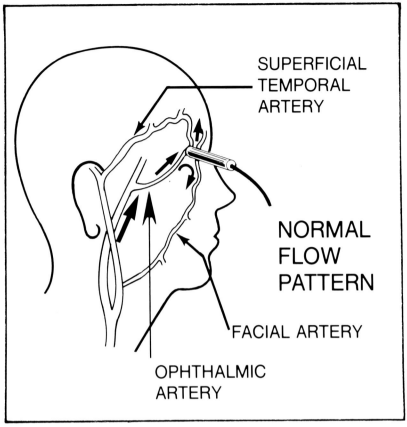

SUPERFICIAL
TEMPORAL
ARTERY

NORMAL
FLOW
PATTERN

FACIAL ARTERY

OPHTHALMIC
ARTERY

Figure 14-1. The anatomy of the branches of the ophthalmic artery and the anastomotic networks.

frontal signal is diminished, this implies collateralization through the circle of Willis, and is again suggestive of significant internal carotid stenosis or occlusion. It is important that carotid compression be performed low in the neck and the bifurcation be avoided. Compression only need be performed for a few seconds. Although this has shown itself to be a safe maneuver when performed as described, it is not used as frequently as the ipsilateral compression techniques.

A flow diagram for the performance and interpretation of periorbital Doppler examination is provided in Figure 14-3.

The frequency of collateral pathways with significant carotid disease has been stated as 64 percent for the superficial temporal, 20 percent for the facial artery, and 7 percent for the contralateral internal carotid.[4]

The diagnostic accuracy of a well-performed periorbital Doppler examination has been quoted as 98 percent in the detection of the presence or absence of a 50-percent or greater stenosis in diameter or occlusion of the internal carotid.[8] If only the supraorbital artery is examined, the diagnostic accuracy falls to 61 percent.[9] It is therefore important to carefully evaluate all possible sources of collateral supply in the performance of this examination.

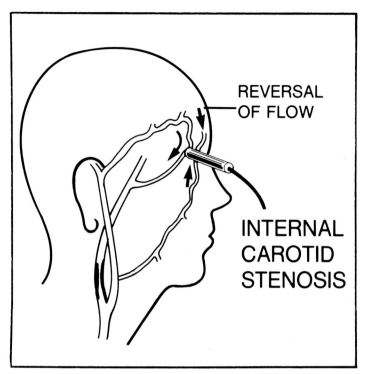

Figure 14-2. Reversal of flow into the orbit seen with significant internal carotid stenosis.

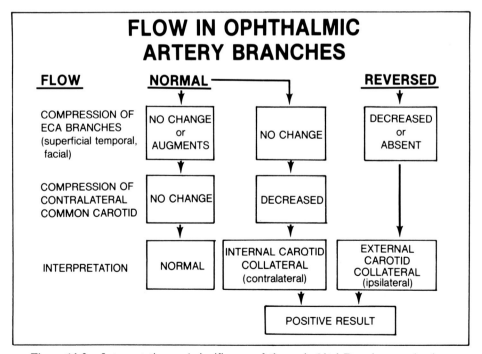

Figure 14-3. Interpretation and significance of the periorbital Doppler examination.

Limitations

Periorbital Doppler examination is useful in the diagnosis of hemodynamically significant (greater than 50 percent of diameter) lesions. It has been shown that more than half of patients with symptomatic operable disease of the internal carotid will have stenoses of less than 40 to 50 percent as demonstrated by arteriography.[10] This examination does not detect nonobstructing lesions of clinical significance.[7,9] Furthermore, the periorbital Doppler examination does not distinguish between a stenotic and an occluded internal carotid artery.

Within the scope of these limitations, the periorbital examination is a useful technique for the screening of patients with asymptomatic bruits, and for the study of those patients with nonhemispheric or equivocal symptoms.

PHOTOPLETHYSMOGRAPHY

The technique of photoplethysmography has been well described.[11] This method detects pulsatile cutaneous blood flow. A probe is used that transmits infrared light, which is then reflected from the microcirculation of the skin. The reflected light is received by an infrared-sensitive phototransistor, which is coupled to an amplifier that provides a graphic output of pulsation. The amplitude of the signal varies with the content of blood in the microcirculation and is normally pulsatile. Probes are placed on the forehead, above the medial aspect of the eyebrow, and in the area supplied by the frontal and supraorbital arteries.

In a normal subject, diminution of pulsation over the supraorbital or frontal areas occurs only with compression of the ipsilateral common carotid artery (Fig. 14-4A). If a significant diminution in pulsation is produced by compression of the superficial temporal, the facial, or the contralateral common carotid arteries, this is diagnostic of significant collateral flow to the internal carotid system, and is interpreted as a positive result (greater than 50-percent stenosis) (Fig. 14-4B,C).

Barnes[12] has stated that the technique of supraorbital photoplethysmography has 100 percent sensitivity in the diagnosis of the presence of a significant lesion in the internal carotid. In his series, 68 of 76 normal carotid arteries were detected (a specificity of 89 percent).

CAROTID PHONOANGIOGRAPHY

The audio and visual analysis of carotid bruits has proved to be a helpful adjunct in the diagnosis of symptomatic carotid stenosis. The presence of an audible bruit in the neck, especially in an elderly patient, is usually an indication of the presence of some degree of stenosis of the internal carotid.

The technique of carotid phonoangiography (CPA) has been well described by Kartchner.[13] With the patient resting comfortably on his or her back, audiofrequency traces are made using a microphone placed over three regions of the neck (as high as possible over the palpable carotid pulse, over the region of the carotid bifurcation, and at the base of the neck). Photographs are taken of the displays of these recordings.

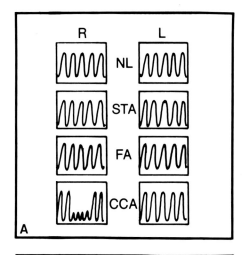
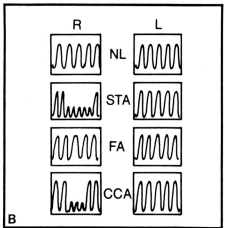
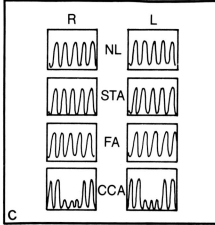

Figure 14-4. (A) Right (R) and left (L) photoplethysmograph tracings normally (NL) and with compression of the superficial temporal (STA), the facial (FA), and the common carotid (CCA) arteries on the right side. Only right CCA compressions decrease pulsation. (B) a decrease in pulsation on the right with STA compression suggests right internal carotid stenosis with collateral flow from the STA. A decrease with right CCA compression is normal. (C) A decrease in pulsation on the right with compression of the left CCA suggests right internal carotid stenosis with collateral flow from the left CCA. A decrease on the left is normal.

The presence of a bruit in the middle or high regions of the neck only suggests that it is of carotid origin.[13] Bruits heard in the low portion of the neck that attenuate or disappear at higher levels are usually of cardiac or great vessel origin. A normal CPA tracing is shown in Fig. 14-5.

In general, a bruit is not detectable until a 30-percent stenosis is present. This will not be audible but will be observable on the tracing of the bruit.[14] As the degree of stenosis increases, the bruit becomes more and more high pitched, extends further into systole, and, in the presence of severe stenosis, extends into diastole. A bruit extending into diastole is diagnostic of internal carotid stenosis. Bruits originating in the external carotid do not have a diastolic component. Figures 14-6 and 14-7 shows CPA tracings from patients with mild and severe degrees of carotid stenosis.

Because the intensity of the bruit is related to size of the lumen, to the velocity, and to the turbulence of blood flow, the bruit may disappear as the stenosis exceeds 80 to 90 percent. Therefore, a high-grade stenosis and an occluded internal carotid may produce a normal tracing. The first heart sound may also be absent from tracings above the lesion.

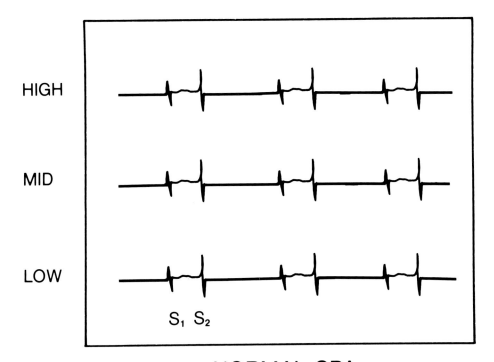

HIGH

MID

LOW

S₁ S₂

NORMAL CPA

Figure 14-5. A normal CPA tracing. No turbulence between heart sounds (S₁, S₂) is noted.

Kartchner and McRae[13] have studied the usefulness of CPA in 200 patients in whom arteriography was performed and have demonstrated that this technique has a sensitivity of 85 percent and a specificity of 88 percent in the detection of a significant stenosis (greater than 50 percent). The total accuracy of CPA was 73 percent.

While lesions as small as a 30 percent reduction in area may produce bruits detectable by CPA, these are not of hemodynamic significance. This technique is applicable to mass screening and follow-up of carotid bruits, and is useful in monitoring the progression of asymptomatic stenoses. However, it is rarely used as the sole technique of carotid evaluation.

OCULOPLETHYSMOGRAPHY—PULSE DELAY

The oculoplethysmograph (OPG) described by Kartchner and McRae[15] measures waveforms in the eyes and ears in an attempt to detect significant internal carotid stenosis. Saline-filled suction cups are applied to each eye (40–50 mm Hg suction), and opacity-sensitive light detectors are attached to each ear. These indirectly represent internal carotid (ophthalmic artery) and external carotid (posterior auricular artery) flow.

The pulsatile signals recorded from each area are amplified and measured for pulse delays. Significant stenosis of one internal carotid will produce a measurable delay between the arrival of the two ocular waveforms. This delay is considered to

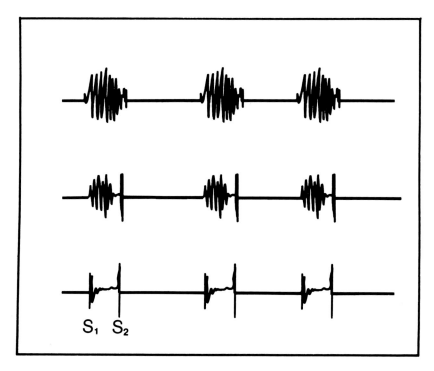

50% STENOSIS OF ICA

Figure 14-6. A 50-percent stenosis of the internal carotid artery. The bruit is most prominent in middle and high neck.

represent significant stenosis or occlusion (Fig. 14-8A,B). A delay between the signals of the two eyes, or between ipsilateral eye and ear (internal versus external carotid) is considered diagnostic.

When used alone, the OPG (pulse delay) has an accuracy of 80 percent in the detection of a significant stenosis of the internal carotid.[6,15] The studies have been used to search for lesions that produce a reduction in diameter of 50 percent. Accuracy is generally higher in the diagnosis of more severe lesions. However, a study that is normal has a high probability of excluding hemodynamically significant carotid disease. This technique is limited in that it does not do well in the detection of bilateral internal carotid stenoses. Lesions that produce a 50-percent reduction in diameter but which leave a residual lumen of 2.5 mm may also not produce a pulse delay, and will often be missed with this technique.[14]

The use of the OPG with an air-filled transducer (Zira OPG) is also common and has been shown to be equally accurate.[16] It has the advantage of being able to be used with the patient supine rather than sitting, and is therefore favored by many vascular laboratories, including our own.

When both OPG and CPA techniques are combined, an overall diagnostic accuracy of 90 percent in the detection of lesions that reduce luminal area by 75 percent can be achieved.[14,16] Severe bilateral disease with bilateral pulse delays in ocular tracings, and smaller lesions that do not produce pulse delays, may be better and more correctly diagnosed with the addition of the CPA data. Again, the combination

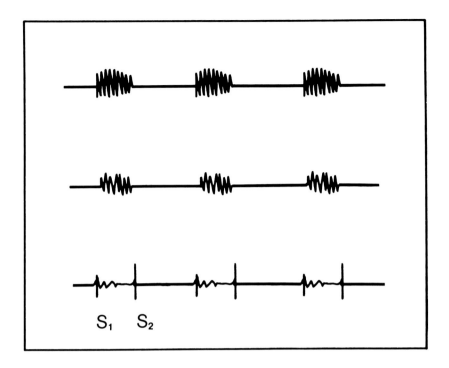

85% STENOSIS OF ICA

Figure 14-7. An 85-percent stenosis of the internal carotid artery. The bruit extends into diastole.

of these techniques is a rapid way to screen for and follow the progression of carotid disease.

OCULOPNEUMOPLETHYSMOGRAPHY

Oculopneumoplethysmography (Gee OPG) attempts to measure internal carotid pressure by studying ophthalmic artery pressure responses to varying amounts of suction placed upon the globe. The technique was developed by Gee, and has been extensively described.[17] Using suction cups applied to the sclera, a vacuum of 500 mm Hg is applied to the globe and gradually reduced. The intraocular pressure thus generated correlates with the suction applied. When the intraocular pressure falls below the systolic pressure in the ophthalmic artery, pulsations measurable on the surface of the globe return, and this is recorded as the ophthalmic artery pressure.

The test is considered to be positive if there is a pressure difference between the eyes greater than 5 mm Hg, if one or both ophthalmic artery pressures fall below a standard regression line given by the formula

$$OAP = 0.4216 \times Brachial\ BP + 38.94$$

or if ophthalmic artery pressures are greater than 140 mm Hg, and there is a difference in pulse amplitude between the eyes. An example of a positive study is seen in Figure 14-9.

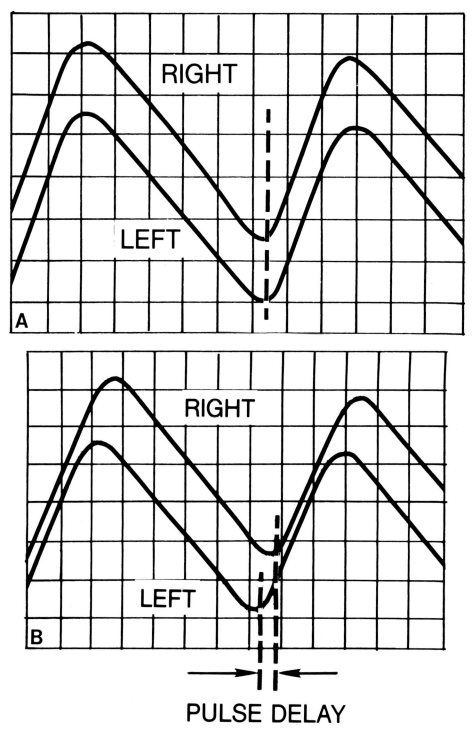

Figure 14-8. (A) Oculoplethysmographic tracings from a normal patient. There is no pulse delay. (B) Tracings from patient with a significant right internal carotid stenosis. Note the pulse delay.

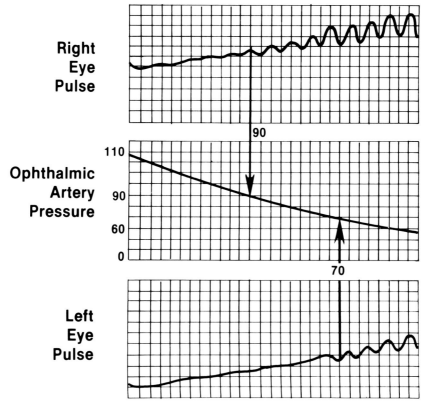

Figure 14-9. An example of a positive Gee OPG. Note the decreased ophthalmic pressure in the left eye, and the pressure gradients between the eyes.

This technique has a 90 to 95-percent accuracy in the detection of a lesion in the internal carotid system that produces a stenosis of more than 50-percent diameter.[17] A potential adjunct in the use of the Gee OPG is in the preoperative measurement of internal carotid back pressure. By maintaining intraocular pressure at 60 mm Hg, the ipsilateral common carotid can be compressed low in the neck. If no pulsations are seen in that globe, then it may be concluded that the collateral flow is such that perfusion pressure is less than 60 mm Hg. This may affect intraoperative decisions regarding the use of a shunt. However, the technique is rarely used in place of intraoperative carotid stump pressures.

Relative contraindications to this technique are recent ocular surgery, a history of retinal detachment, and uncontrolled glaucoma. This technique is highly accurate, and is valuable in the assessment of carotid disease at a functional level.

SPECTRAL PHONONAGIOGRAPHY

The technique of spectral analysis of carotid bruits described by Lees[18] is a newer technique that has shown itself to be accurate in the evaluation of actual lumen size in the internal carotid system. Using a standard microphone, CPA tracings are obtained and subjected to spectral analysis using fast Fourier transform. In the resultant display of the spectrum of a bruit, (a plot of intensity versus frequency), a "break frequency" (that frequency above which the intensity drops sharply) can be discerned (Fig. 14-10). The residual lumen of the vessel being studied (in millimeters) is determined as 500 divided by the break frequency in Hertz.

$$d = 500/f_o$$

In an analysis of 31 bifurcations in 33 patients, this technique was able to predict lumen diameter to within 0.5 mm of that measured in the surgical specimen.[18] This technique is new and promising. Its accuracy appears high, and it may well become more important in the future.

The major limitation is that if a bruit is too faint to hear, it cannot be adequately subjected to frequency analysis. There also is a considerable amount of experience necessary for an accurate evaluation.

SUMMARY

It must be stressed that the techniques discussed here are not designed to detect plaque disease, or lesions that do not cause a significant hemodynamic derangement. Other techniques, such as real-time Duplex imaging (combining B-mode ultrasound

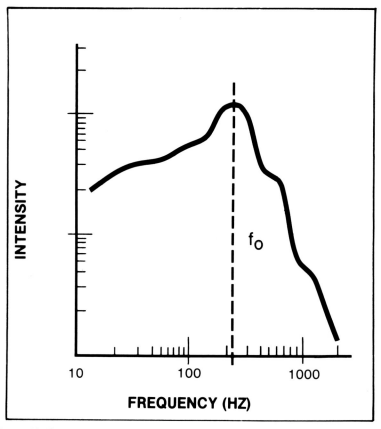

Figure 14-10. A spectral display of a bruit, plotting intensity versus frequency.

and Doppler spectral analysis) and digital subtraction angiography are better suited to the detection of these lesions, and will be discussed in another chapter.

The methods of examination of the carotid system presented here are rapid, simple, painless, and accurate in the diagnosis of significant hemodynamic lesions. While no one method is clearly superior, a combination of these techniques will increase the total diagnostic accuracy.[12,14,17,19,20,21] They provide a convenient way to follow patients with asymptomatic bruits, to study and follow the course of stenotic lesions, and to diagnose the presence or absence of hemodynamically significant lesions in patients with vague or nonlocalized complaints.

A proper understanding of the nature of the information provided by these noninvasive tests permits them to be quite helpful in patient management. In the symptomatic patient in whom the noninvasive studies do not demonstrate a hemodynamically significant stenotic lesion, angiography is still necessary to rule out the diagnosis of plaque disease. Operative correction can then be performed if deemed appropriate. Asymptomatic patients with hemodynamically significant stenoses may be evaluated and followed with these techniques with an eye toward further evaluation or surgical correction if the stenosis progresses or symptoms develop. Within the limitations discussed, the techniques for noninvasive diagnosis and screening allow the clinician to make more rational decisions about the management of carotid artery disease.

REFERENCES

1. Stallones RA, Dyken ML, Fang HCH, et al: Report of the joint committee for stroke facilities. Stroke 3:360–371, 1972

2. Baker WH: The asymptomatic carotid bruit, in Baker WH (ed): Diagnosis and Treatment of Carotid Artery Disease. Mount Kisco, NY, Futura Publishing, 1979, pp 131–136

3. Baker WH: Hemispheric cerebrovascular insufficiency, in Baker WH (ed): Diagnosis and Treatment of Carotid Artery Disease. Mount Kisco, NY, Futura Publishing, 1979, pp 115–123

4. Fields WS, North RR, Hass WK, et al: Joint study of extracranial arterial occlusion as a cause of stroke. I: Organization of a study and survey of patient population. JAMA 203:955–960, 1968

5. Hass WK, Fields WS, North RR, et al: Joint study of extracranial arterial occlusion. II: Arteriography, technique, sites, complications. JAMA 203:961–968, 1968

6. Kartchner MM, McRae LP, Crain V, et al: Oculoplethysmography: An adjunct to arteriography in the diagnosis of extracranial carotid occlusive disease. Am J Surg 132:728–732, 1976

7. Brockenbrough EC: Periorbital Doppler velocity evaluation of carotid obstruction, in Bernstein EF (ed): Noninvasive Diagnostic Techniques in Vascular Disease. St. Louis, C.V. Mosby, 1982, pp 231–247

8. Barnes RW, Russell HE, Bone GE, et al: Doppler cerebrovascular examination: Improved results with refinements in technique. Stroke 8:468–471, 1977

9. Lye CR, Sumner DS, Strandness DE Jr: The accuracy of the supraorbital Doppler examination in the diagnosis of hemodynamically significant carotid occlusive disease. Surgery 79:42–45, 1976

10. Eisenberg RL, Menzek WR, Moore WS: Relationship of transient ischemic attacks and angiographically demonstrable lesions of the carotid artery. Stroke 8:483–486, 1977

11. Barnes RW, Clayton JM, Bone GE, et al: Supraorbital photoplethysmography—simple accurate screening for carotid occlusive disease. J Surg Res 22:319–327, 1977

12. Barnes RW, Garrett WV, Slaymaker EE, et al: Doppler ultrasound and supraorbital photoplethysmography for noninvasive screening of carotid occlusive disease. Am J Surg 134:183–186, 1977

13. Kartchner MM, McRae LP: Auscultation for carotid bruits in cerebrovascular insufficiency. JAMA 210:494–497, 1969

14. McRae LP, Kartchner MM: Oculoplethysmography: Timed comparison of ocular

pulses and carotid phonoangiography, in Bernstein EF (ed): Noninvasive Diagnostic Techniques in Vascular Disease. St. Louis, C. V. Mosby, 1982, pp 87–103

15. Kartchner MM, McRae LP, Morrison FD: Noninvasive detection and evaluation of carotid occlusive disease. Arch Surg 106:528–535, 1973

16. Malone JM, Bean B, Laguna J, et al: Diagnosis of carotid artery stenosis comparison of oculoplethysmography and Doppler supraorbital examination. Ann Surg 191:347–354, 1979

17. Gee W, Oller DW, Amundsen DG, et al: The asymptomatic carotid bruit and the ocular pneumoplethysmograph. Arch Surg 112:1381–1388, 1977

18. Kistler JP, Lees RS, Miller A, et al: Corre-

lation of spectral phonoangiography and carotid angiography with gross pathology in carotid stenosis. N Engl J Med 305:417–419, 1981

19. Gross WS, Verta MJ Jr, Van Bellen B, et al: Comparison of noninvasive diagnostic techniques in carotid artery occlusive disease. Surg 82:271–278, 1977

20. Kartchner MM, McRae LP: Noninvasive evaluation and management of the "asymptomatic" carotid bruit. Surgery 82:840–847, 1977

21. McDonald PT, Rich NM, Collins GJ, et al: Doppler cerebrovascular examination, oculoplethysmography, and ocular pneumoplethysmography. Use in detection of carotid disease: A prospective clinical trial. Arch Surg 113:1341–1349, 1978

Joel Leland

15
Ultrasound of the Carotid Arteries

Major cerebral vascular accidents, which are frequently preceded by transient ischemic attacks, are often secondary to carotid occlusive disease. Atherosclerotic lesions of the carotid artery, at or near the bifurcation, can cause symptoms from a reduction in cerebral blood flow resulting from stenosis or occlusion of the internal carotid or intracranial ischemia resulting from emboli from lacerating intimal plaques.[1]

A majority of patients who have suffered a cerebral vascular accident have a surgically accessible obstructing lesion in the carotid bifurcation or the proximal internal carotid artery.[2]

Currently, angiography is the only procedure available for definitive diagnosis of the site and distribution of atheromatous plaques and for diagnosing stenosis of the carotid arteries. It is, however, an invasive technique that is potentially hazardous, and it may underestimate the extent of the pathologic condition.

A noninvasive technique that is safe and accurate would clearly be a useful tool in the diagnosis of carotid occlusive disease. During the last few years a number of noninvasive tests have been developed in an attempt to provide an alternative to angiography or as screening procedures. Oculoplethysmography,[3,4] carotid phonoangiography,[5] and pulsed Doppler[6,7] have become standard techniques in many vascular laboratories.

Oculoplethysmography, using the technique of Kartchner or Gee, has given excellent results in the diagnosis of unilateral carotid stenosis.[3,4] It is an indirect measure of cerebral vascular flow, however, and is less accurate with bilateral carotid disease.

Bruits heard over the carotid bifurcation can be analyzed by phonoangiography. A loud bruit, however, may be associated with a minimal stenosis and the reduced blood flow associated with marked stenosis may not be sufficient to cause a bruit.[8] Phonoangiography together with oculoplethysmography has an accuracy of 89 percent in diagnosing a stenosis of greater than 40 percent.[9]

Ultrasonic B-scanning is a good screening test because it provides an image of

IMAGING OF THE PERIPHERAL VASCULAR SYSTEM Copyright © 1984 by Grune & Stratton.
ISBN 0-8089-1636-X

the vessels. Early work with conventional B-scanners yielded poor results because of poor resolution.[10,11] However, the recent development of high resolution transducers in the 7–10 MHz range has improved studies. These transducers, with their decreased penetration but high resolution, are ideally suited for the study of the superficially located carotid artery.

High-frequency gray scale ultrasonography reliably outlines the extent and severity of atheromatous plaques and demonstrates stenosis in the common carotid artery and its bifurcation vessels.[12] Green[13] and Mercier et al.[14] have reported satisfactory high-resolution images using a 10 MHz transducer with a real-time B-scanner.

An overall accuracy of 70 percent using ultrasonic imaging has been reported.[2] In a series of 19 patients reported by Gompels et al.,[15] all stenoses greater than 30 percent were detected. Plaques were demonstrated in the arteries. The accuracy of B-scanning can be increased by combining it with pulsed Doppler, ultrasound.

Scanning is performed with a patient in a supine position. A pillow is placed under the shoulders with the neck held in extension, and the head rotated away from the side being scanned.

Real-time ultrasound allows greater flexibility than static B-scanning. With real-time ultrasound, the ultrasonographer is easily able to find the proper scanning planes. Initially palpating the carotid artery is helpful in assessing the course of the vessel in the neck. The transducer is then placed over the expected course of the artery, usually just medial to the sternocleidomastoid.

The use of several types of real-time units has been reported. These include linear array systems with a 7-MHz transducer,[16] and the new "small parts" scanners with a 10-MHz transducer.[2,15] All these units employ high-resolution transducers of low penetrance. Scans are obtained in longitudinal and transverse planes.

With real-time ultrasound scanning, the arteries are identified by their pulsatile nature. Arteries with a smooth internal lining and an echo-free lumen are considered normal (Fig. 15-1). The common carotid normally widens at the bulb just proximal to the bifurcation. The internal carotid is more readily demonstrated by ultrasound than is the external carotid, since it tends to follow the course of the common carotid artery. The internal carotid has a more posterior course than the external carotid, but, with proper alignment of the transducer, the internal carotid and the external carotid can be seen in one scanning plane in most patients (Fig. 15-2). On transverse scans, the external carotid artery lies anteromedial to the internal carotid and is usually of a smaller caliber (Fig. 15-3).

Ectasia of the aortic arch secondary to arteriosclerosis produces an elongated and elevated arch, which can push the innominate and right common carotid arteries upward. This will produce buckling of the carotid artery and a pulsatile mass that is indistinguishable from an aneurysm on palpation. This pseudoaneurysm effect can be distinguished from a true aneurysm by careful real-time scanning, which shows an ectatic but otherwise normal carotid artery and obviates the need for further work-up (Fig. 15-4A,B).

Atherosclerotic plaques are identified as echogenic structures within the lumen of the vessel (Fig. 15-5). Intimal irregularities and intramural filling defects were interpreted as atheromatous plaques (Fig. 15-6). Only those abnormalities that could be reproduced were considered abnormal, since reverberations may produce artifacts. The anteroposterior diameter of a narrowed section was measured and compared with

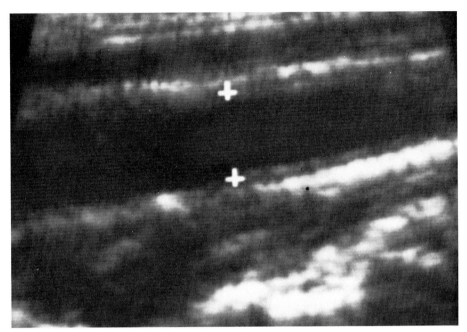

Figure 15-1. A normal common carotid artery with a smooth internal lining and echo-free lumen.

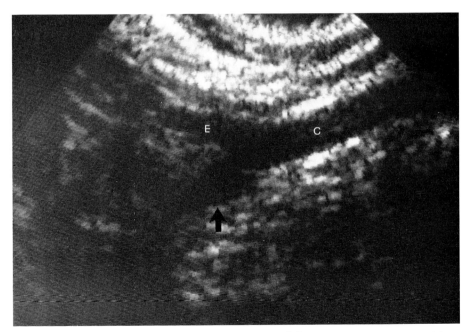

Figure 15-2. Bifurcation of the common carotid artery (C) into the external carotid (E) and the more posterior internal carotid (arrow).

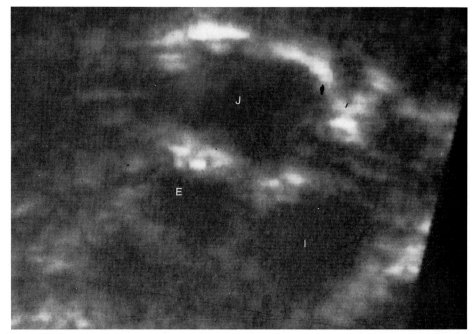

Figure 15-3. Transverse scan just above the bifurcation showing the jugular vein (J) and internal (I) and external (E) carotid arteries.

a normal section of carotid artery and a ratio representing the percentage of stenosis of approximately 40 percent was derived (Fig. 15-7).

Abnormalities of the carotid system other than plaques and stenosis have been described. Aneurysms can be detected as echo-free saccular or cystlike lesions in continuity with the carotid artery. An echo-free cystlike lesion demonstrating expansile pulsations is diagnostic of an aneurysm. However, a large aneurysm fed by a small artery may show little pulsation.[16]

Carotid body tumors, which are neoplasms of the chemoreceptors of the carotid body, situated at the bifurcation have been described. Solid, well-circumscribed, but weakly echogenic masses at the bifurcation are diagnostic.[17] Carotid artery thrombus, which is a rare condition, can also be detected.[18]

There are currently several limitations to the ultrasonic imaging of the carotid arteries. Vessels with calcification in the anterior wall create problems because of the large acoustic interfaces presented to the ultrasonic beam. Further penetration beyond the calcified area is prevented, causing an acoustic shadow that makes visualization of the lumen impossible, thereby preventing assessment of any narrowing of the lumen (Fig. 15-8). If the plaque arises from the deep or posterior wall, then the narrowing can be assessed. Ultrasound has also been found to be ineffective in certain circumstances in quantitating the actual degree of obstruction.[12,19] It has also been shown to be inaccurate for total occlusions.[20]

Other limitations include the inability to detect ulcerative plaques that are the source of transient ischemic attacks.[10,12,19] It has also been found difficult to distinguish a noncalcified plaque or fresh thrombus from blood by B-mode scanning.[7] This is because of the inability of ultrasound to differentiate between substances of similar

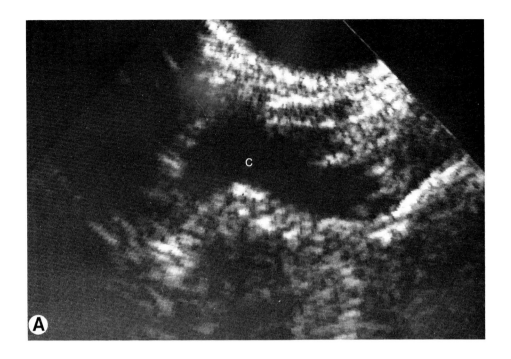

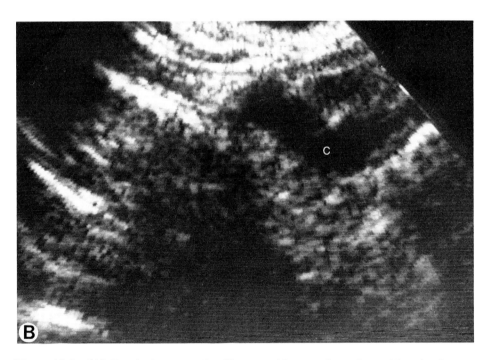

Figure 15-4. (A) Ectatic but normal caliber carotid artery in patient with pulsatile mass suggesting an aneurysm. (B) Tortuous carotid artery. Longitudinal scans of ectatic common carotid (C) arteries in two patients. Both had pulsatile neck masses.

291

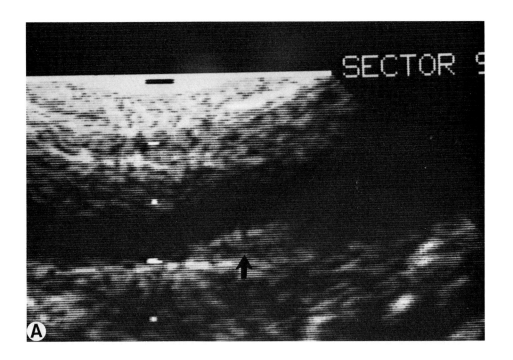

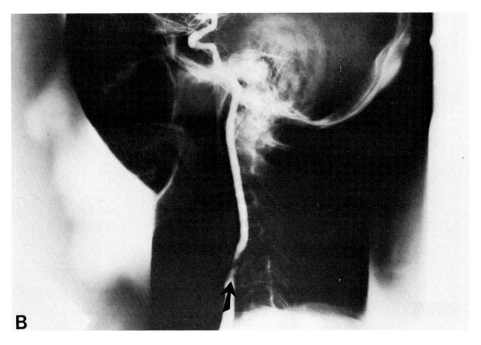

Figure 15-5. (A) An echogenic mass (atherosclerotic plaque, arrow) in the posterior aspect of the common carotid artery. (B) An arteriogram confirming the ultrasonic findings (arrow).

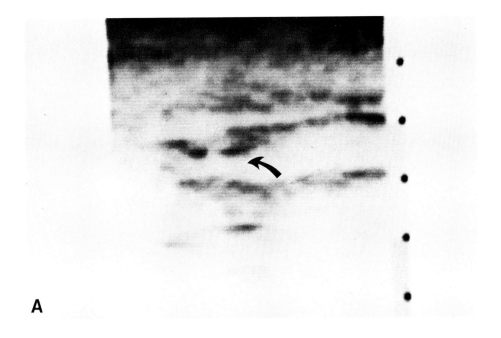

A

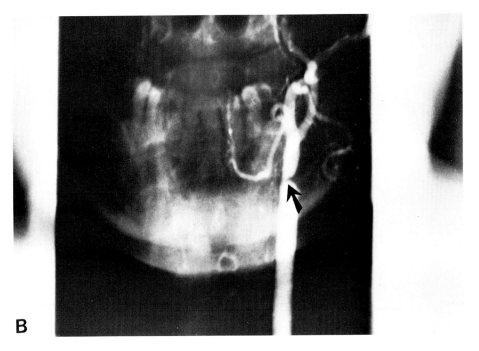

B

Figure 15-6. (A) An intraluminal filling defect (arrow) with 50-percent narrowing of the lumen of the common carotid artery. (B) An arteriogram of the same patient.

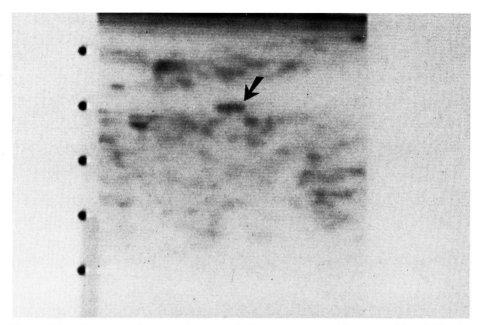

Figure 15-7. Plaque on the posterior wall of the common carotid artery with calcification (arrow) demonstrating acoustic shadowing. The lumen is narrowed 40 percent.

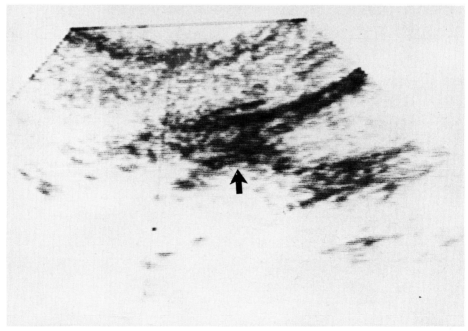

Figure 15-8. Calcified plaque on the anterior wall of the common carotid artery obscuring the lumen of the vessel (arrow).

acoustic impedance. Therefore, a totally occluded vessel may appear normal by ultrasound if the thrombus is fresh.

Further studies along with refinement of the equipment should help overcome these limitations. At the present time, the addition of pulsed Doppler ultrasound can increase the accuracy of ultrasonic imaging of the carotid system.

High-frequency gray scale ultrasonic imaging is relatively sensitive in identifying the presence of stenosis, but currently is insensitive in its ability to assess the degree of stenosis. It is also unable to delineate ulceration. Ultrasound does appear to be useful as a screening test in cerebrovascular disease, especially in combination with pulsed Doppler, which would help rule out areas of stenosis missed on B-scans.

Presently, a normal real-time ultrasonic B-scan of the carotid artery is a strong indication of patency of the vessel and would militate against further invasive procedures. Further refinement is necessary, however, to identify those patients who are candidates for arteriography. With further developments in technology, the clinical application of ultrasonic imaging will increase.

REFERENCES

1. Moore WS, Hall AD: Importance of emboli from carotid bifurcation in pathogenesis of cerebral ischemic attacks. Arch Surg 101:708, 1970

2. Humber PR, Leopold GR, Wickbom IG, et al: Ultrasonic imaging of the carotid arterial system. Am J Surg 140:199–202, 1980

3. Kartchner MM, McRae LP, Crain V, et al: Oculoplethysmography: An adjunct to arteriography in diagnosis of extracranial carotid occlusive disease. Am J Surg 132:728–732, 1976

4. Gee W, Mehigan JT, Wylie EJ: Measurement of collateral hemispheric blood pressure by ocular pneumoplethysmography. Am J Surg 130:121–127, 1975

5. Kartchner MM, McRae LP, Morrison FP: Noninvasive detection and evaluation of carotid occlusive disease. Arch Surg 106:528, 1973

6. Barnes RW: Doppler ultrasonic arteriography and flow velocity analysis in carotid artery disease, in Bernstein E.F. (ed): Non-invasive Diagnostic Techniques in Vascular Disease. St. Louis, C.V. Mosby, 1978

7. Blackslear WM, Phillips DJ, Thiele BL, et al: Detection of carotid occlusive disease by ultrasonic imaging and pulsed Doppler spectrum analysis. Surgery 86:698–706, 1979

8. McRae LP, Kartchner MM: Oculoplethysmography: Timed comparison of occular pulses and carotid phonoangiography, in Bernstein E.F. (ed): Non-Invasive Diagnostic Technique in Vascular Disease. St. Louis, C.V. Mosby, 1978

9. Kartchner MM, McRae LP: Noninvasive evaluation and management of the asymptomatic carotid bruit. Surgery 82:840–847, 1977

10. Clinger C: Ultrasonic carotid echoarteriography. AJR 106:282–295, 1969

11. Anderson R, Powell D, Litak J: B-mode sonography as a screening procedure for asymptomatic carotid bruits. AJR 124:292–296, 1975

12. Cooperberg PL, Robertson WD, Fry P, et al: High resolution real time ultrasound of the carotid bifurcation. J Clin Ultrasound 7:13–17, 1979

13. Green PS: Real time high resolution ultrasonic carotid arteriography system, in Bernstein EF (ed): Noninvasive Diagnostic Technique in Vascular Disease. St. Louis, C.V. Mosby, 1978, pp 23–39

14. Mercier LA, Greenleaf JF, Evans TC, et al: High resolution ultrasound arteriography: A comparison with carotid angiography, in Bernstein EF (ed): Non-invasive Diagnostic Technique in Vascular Disease. St. Louis, C.V. Mosby, 1978, pp 231–244

15. Gompels BM: High definition imaging of carotid arteries using a standard commercial ultrasound "B" scanner. Br J Radiol 52:608–619, 1979

16. Yeh HC, Mitty HA, Wolf BS, et al: Ultrasound of the brachiocephalic arteries. Radiology 132:403–408, 1979

17. Gooding FAW: Gray scale ultrasound detection of carotid body tumor. Radiology 132:409–410, 1979

18. Dunnick NR, Schuette WH, Shawker TR: Ultrasonic demonstration of thrombus in the common carotid artery. AJR 133:544–545, 1979

19. Leopold GR: Ultrasonography of superficially located structures. Radiol Clin North Am 18:161–172, 1980

20. Hobson RW, Silvia MB, Katocs AS, et al: Comparison of pulsed Doppler and real time B-mode echo arteriography for non-invasive imaging of the extracranial carotid arteries. Surgery 87:286–293, 1980

Steven Pinsky

16

Radionuclide Evaluation of the Carotid Arteries

TECHNIQUE

The radionuclide evaluation of the carotid arteries is usually performed as part of a radionuclide brain scan. Radionuclide angiography of any type must be performed with a scintillation camera rather than a rectilinear scanner. The dynamic portion of brain scans is generally performed in either the anterior or vertex positions. If there is a possibility of a pathologic condition in the carotid arteries, the study should be performed in the anterior position. For the best visualization of the carotid arteries, the patient is positioned with the neck extended and the field of view slightly lower than when the area of interest is the intracranial vessels. Moody et al.,[1] suggested performing the procedure with the patient supine with bolsters under the shoulders so that the head could be extended as far as possible and the detector centered over the thyroid cartilage. We prefer having the patient in a seated position with the neck extended. The radionuclide of choice would be the one used for the radionuclide brain scan. At most institutions this is either ^{99m}Tc-pertechnetate, ^{99m}Tc-DTPA, or ^{99m}Tc-glucoheptonate. The usual dose is 15 to 20 mCi, and it is important that this be in a volume of 1 ml or less. The high specific activity is important in obtaining a good bolus injection. The radionuclide is injected at the antecubital fossa, preferably in the brachial vein, using the technique of Oldendorf et al.[2] This consists of using a blood pressure cuff inflated to a pressure between systolic and diastolic pressures. The cuff is placed above the site of injection of the radionuclide and is rapidly removed after injection to produce a good bolus of activity. An alternative technique involves the use of a three-way stopcock with the injection of the radionuclide bolus through one valve and the injection of saline through a second valve immediately after the radionuclide is injected. This produces a good bolus of radioactivity. Either of these techniques will give good quality images of the carotid arteries. The images are recorded on x-ray or 35-mm film every 2 seconds following the arrival of the bolus on the screen of the persistence scope (Fig. 16-1).

IMAGING OF THE PERIPHERAL VASCULAR SYSTEM Copyright © 1984 by Grune & Stratton.
ISBN 0-8089-1636-X

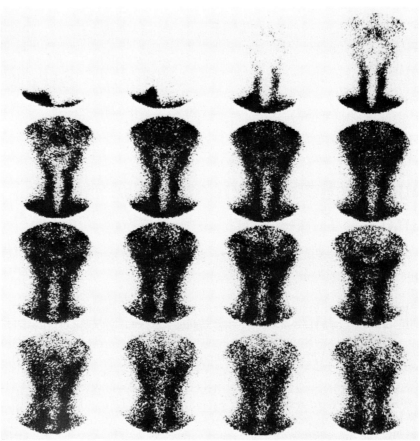

Figure 16-1. A normal carotid angiogram following bolus intravenous injection of ^{99m}Tc-DTPA. Views were obtained every 2 seconds with the neck extended.

Quantitative information may be obtained with the use of a dedicated nuclear medicine computer. The sensitivity of the carotid nuclide angiogram has been shown to increase with the use of the computer (Fig. 16-2). Weissman, et al.[3] demonstrated that the quantitative analysis of the radionuclide angiogram increased the sensitivity for both unilateral and bilateral carotid stenosis. They found that by comparing the slopes of the activity curves over the carotid vessels, they could detect both total and subtotal occlusions. Their study found other measurements to be less reliable.

Quantitation of carotid flow has been particularly helpful in patients undergoing serial studies. This is frequently performed on patients who are to undergo surgery to improve their carotid circulation. The extended position of the neck allows visualization of that region of the carotids that is most accessible to surgical correction. This is the area close to the carotid bifurcation. Winston and Cohen[4] reported that by using ECG-gated studies of carotid arterial pulsation, they were able to achieve 94-percent sensitivity for the detection of arterial narrowing in patients with narrowing of the carotid artery that was 50 percent or greater.

In the visual evaluation of carotid flow, one area of potentially misleading information is the horizontal void representing the absorption of energy by the overlying

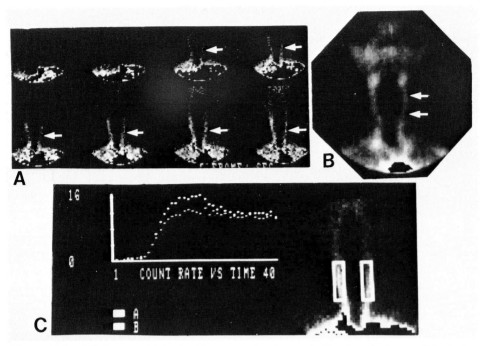

Figure 16-2. (A) Images obtained with a computer demonstrating flow in the carotid arteries showing decreased flow in the left carotid (arrow). (B) Images show slightly decreased flow to the left carotid (double arrow). (C) Quantitative study with areas of interest over the carotids demonstrates a quantitative difference in flow between the right carotid and left carotid.

mandible. This will appear as a focal area of reduced uptake involving both carotids. While the common carotid artery is normally easy to palpate, and auscultation of the neck to detect carotid bruits is a commonly employed procedure, a negative physical finding in patients with severe carotid artery disease is not unusual.[5,6]

When another pathologic condition in the carotid arteries is suspected, such as an aneurysm, static imaging of the carotid vessels is advised. This is best performed with technetium-labeled red cells.[7] The technique for labeling red blood cells is discussed in the chapter on radionuclide angiography. The advantage of static blood pool images is that they allow views to be taken in several positions, and higher count images can be obtained so that an abnormality such as an occlusion can be best seen (Fig. 16-3). The clinical diagnosis of aneurysm is confirmed when there is early filling of radioactivity during the arterial phase in the same region that has an increased blood pool on the static images (Fig. 16-4).

CLINICAL INDICATIONS

The most common carotid pathologic condition is atherosclerotic narrowing. The flow study is a useful screening procedure, and when a computer is used, quantitative evaluation confirms abnormal flow in the carotids. With occlusion of greater than 80 percent of one common or internal carotid artery, the radionuclide angiogram will

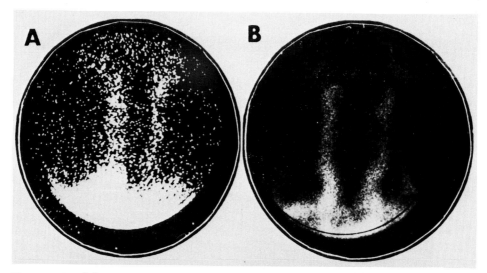

Figure 16-3. (A) Flow study using Technetium-DTPA show relatively decreased flow on the left. (B) Images obtained with labeled red cells and static views give a better impression of decreased flow in the left carotid.

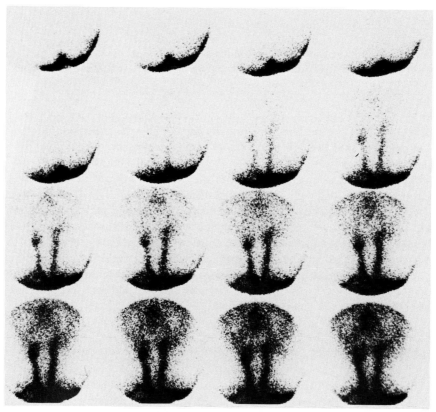

Figure 16-4. Flow study demonstrating a small aneurysm in the upper portion of the right carotid artery. Widening is noted in the arterial phase. It is difficult to evaluate widening in the later views because of the overlap of the venous structures.

demonstrate diminished perfusion through the artery or in the ipsilateral cerebral hemisphere in 80 to 90 percent of patients. Patients with less than 50 percent stenosis are not detected by this technique. Griep et al.[8] found that with visual analysis of the radionuclide angiograms, complete carotid occlusions were detected in 11 of 14 patients, while partial stenoses of 50 to 80 percent were detected in 3 of 6 patients. They were particularly disappointed with the results in bilateral carotid stenosis. Cowan et al.[9] demonstrated that 64 percent of 22 patients with significant carotid disease had abnormal dynamic studies. Two of these patients had bilateral carotid disease that was not detected. Wise et al.[10] suggested that radionuclide angiogram would detect 75 percent of carotid artery obstructions that were confirmed by angiography.

Mishkin and Dyken[11] suggested that obstruction of an internal carotid artery would result in increased radionuclide activity on the angiographic phase in the nasopharyngeal area. They labeled this finding the "hot nose" sign (Fig. 16-5). Atheroslerotic disease in the extracranial portion of the carotid arteries is a frequent yet potentially preventable cause of stroke.[12] Therefore, patients with suspected carotid artery disease detected by either physical examination or by symptoms such as recurrent transient ischemic attacks should be considered for evaluation.

Serafini and Weinstein[13] demonstrated early uptake in a carotid body tumor using ^{99m}Tc-pertechnetate. This early uptake reflected the highly vascular nature of this tumor. They recommended the use of radionuclide angiograms for evaluating family members of patients with carotid body tumors, since this condition has a significant hereditary tendency, being an autosomal-dominant trait. This technique is safe for preoperative evaluation and postoperative follow-up. Peters et al.[14] demonstrated that carotid body chemodectomas can be detected if the increased uptake at the bifurcation in patients with this condition is noted. They advise that this technique can be used as a simple screening procedure for patients suspected of having a chemodectoma and used to differentiate this condition from other masses in the neck such as bronchial cysts, subsalivary tumors, and cervical lymphadenopathy.[14] Laird et al.[15] reported on seven cases of carotid body tumors studied by radionuclide angiography of the carotids. The radionuclide study proved safer than contrast angiography and more reliable than clinical examination. They recommended the nuclear angiogram as the method of choice in the primary screening of patients with suspected carotid-body and glomus-

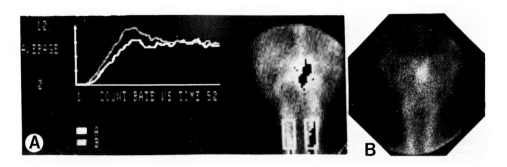

Figure 16-5. (A) Obstruction of the right internal carotid artery on a computer generated image with decreased flow in the right carotid compared with the left demonstrated by the curves of the images. The "hot nose" sign on the delayed view as a result of a change in the normal flow pattern.

jugulare tumors. DeBlanc and Chretien,[16] however, demonstrated that angiofibromas are clinically indistinguishable from carotid body tumors. Moreover, Stevens and Mishkin[17] demonstrated that cervical lymphadenitis may cause increased perfusion from branches of the ipsilateral subclavian artery. This could be mistaken for either a pathologic entity on that side of the neck or contralateral carotid stenosis.

NEW DEVELOPMENTS

A totally different technique was described by Mettinger et al.[18] who have studied iodinated fibrinogen for the detection of atherosclerotic plaques in the carotid arteries. They have used ^{123}I-labeled fibrinogen, which has good imaging properties but is not commercially available. They did demonstrate increased activity over arteriosclerotic regions of vessels in some cases of cerebral ischemia.

Lees et al.[19] demonstrated localization of autologous plasma low-density lipoproteins labeled with iodine-125 in atherosclerotic lesions in the carotid arteries of the neck. The radiopharmaceutical was administered intravenously, and images were obtained 6 to 36 hours after injection. The carotid lesions were imaged successfully in all 3 patients, and the lesions were confirmed by contrast angiography. This technique has great potential if the pharmaceutical can be easily prepared and labeled with either iodine-123 or technetium-99m.

CONCLUSIONS

The image resolution of the radionuclide carotid angiogram is not comparable to that of contrast angiography. There is a low count density in these procedures that significantly effects the resolution. This procedure, however, is noninvasive, while contrast angiography is not without morbidity and mortality. Besides being noninvasive, the radionuclide carotid angiogram offers the advantage of being a relatively good screening procedure that can be performed in conjunction with radionuclide brain scanning with no additional cost or radiation dose to the patient. As a screening procedure, radionuclide angiography has proven useful, particularly with computer processing of the data. The future role, however, must be evaluated in view of the development of digital substraction radiography.

REFERENCES

1. Moody D, Matin P, Goodwin DA: An improved method for visualizing carotid blood flow in the neck. J Nucl Med 12:520–522, 1972

2. Oldendorf WH, Kitano M, Shimizu S: Evaluation of a simple technique for abrupt intravenous injection of an isotope. J Nucl Med 6:205–209, 1965

3. Weissman BN, Holman L, Rosenblum AW: Radionuclide angiography in graded carotid stenosis. Radiology 115:399–402, 1975

4. Winston MA, Cohen SN: ECG-gated blood pool study of carotid arterial pulsation as a sign of stenosis. J Nucl Med 24: 470–474, 1983

5. Toole JF, Patel AN (eds): Cerebrovascular Disease, (ed 2). New York, McGraw-Hill, 1974, pp 123–129

6. Thompson J: Surgery for Cerebrovascular Insufficiency. Springfield, Charles C Thomas, 1968, pp 10–28

7. Ryo UY, Pinsky SM: Radionuclide angiog-

raphy with 99m-Technetium-RBCs. CRC Crit Rev Clin Radiol Nucl Med 8:107–128, 1976

8. Griep RJ, Wise G, Marty R: Detection of carotid obstruction by intravenous radionuclide angiography. Radiology 107:311–316, 1970

9. Cowan RJ, Maynard CD, Meshan I, et al: Value of the routine use of cerebral dynamic radioisotope study. Radiology 107:111–121, 1973

10. Wise G, Brockenbrough EC, Marty R, et al: The detection of carotid artery obstruction: A correlation with arteriography. Stroke 2:105–113, 1971

11. Mishkin FS, Dyken ML: Increased early radionuclide activity in the nasopharyngeal area in patients with internal carotid artery obstruction "hot nose." Radiology 96:77–80, 1970

12. Bauer RB, Meyer JS, Fields WS, et al: Joint study of extracranial arterial occlusion. JAMA 208:509–518, 1969

13. Serafini AN, Weinstein MB: Radionuclide evaluation of a carotid body tumor. J Nucl Med 13:640–643, 1972

14. Peters JL, Ward MW, Fisher C: Diagnosis of carotid body chemodectomia with dynamic radionuclide perfusion scanning. Am J Surg 139:661–664, 1979

15. Laird JD, Ferguson WR, McIlrath, et al: Radionuclide angiography as the primary investigation in chemodectoma. J Nucl Med 24:475–478, 1983

16. DeBlanc HJ, Chretien P: Angiofibroma clinically indistinguishable from carotid body tumor. A possible embryologic relationship. Am J Surg 119:743–745, 1970

17. Stevens JS, Mishkin FS: Abnormal radionuclide angiogram in cervical lymphadenitis. J Nucl Med 17:26, 1976

18. Mettinger KL, Ericson K, Larson S, et al: Detection of atherosclerotic plaques in carotid arteries by the use of I-123-fibrinogen. Lancet 1:242–244, 1978

19. Lees RS, Lees AM, Strauss HW: External imaging of human atherosclerosis. J Nucl Med 24:154–156, 1983

Dushyant V. Patel

17
Arteriography of the Vessels of the Neck

Arteriography is the imaging modality of choice for definitive and accurate diagnosis of vascular abnormalities. The first section of this chapter deals with the techniques, indications, and complications of brachiocephalic (cerebral) arteriography. The second section contains a brief description of the radiographic arterial anatomy, anatomic variants, and common congenital anomalies of the extracranial brachiocephalic arteries. The final section describes common lesions that affect the cervical carotid, the cervical vertebral, and the proximal subclavian arteries.

INDICATIONS, TECHNIQUES, AND COMPLICATIONS OF BRACHIOCEPHALIC ARTERIOGRAPHY

Indications

With continued wider use of cranial computed tomography, the indications for cerebral arteriography have decreased. The more common indications for brachiocephalic arteriography are evaluation of transient ischemic attacks affecting the carotid and vertebral-basilar arteries; diagnosis of head and neck aneurysms and vascular malformations; definition of the vascular anatomy in patients with stroke caused by occlusive vascular disease to guide further treatment; preoperative evaluation or diagnostic confirmation of head and neck masses; evaluation of suspected traumatic injury to extracranial and, less commonly, intracranial vessels; confirmation of stenosis or occlusion suspected by noninvasive techniques in patients with a bruit in the neck about to undergo major thoracic, cardiac, or abdominal surgery (patients with severe asymptomatic carotid occlusive lesions may suffer a stroke from intraoperative hypotension[1]); confirmation of clinical suspicion of a subclavian steal syndrome.

IMAGING OF THE PERIPHERAL VASCULAR SYSTEM Copyright © 1984 by Grune & Stratton.
ISBN   0-8089-1636-X

Contraindications

There are no absolute contraindications to brachiocephalic arteriography. The incidence of reactions to intraarterial injections of contrast media is much lower than that of intravenous injections. In patients with a history of reaction to contrast media, pretreatment with prednisone and diphenhydramine has greatly reduced the risk.[2]

Technique

The first carotid arteriogram was done by Egas Moniz in 1927 by percutaneous needle puncture of the carotid artery.[3] Subsequently, techniques for percutaneous puncture of the vertebral and brachial arteries were introduced. In 1953, Seldinger first described percutaneous introduction of a catheter, which gradually evolved into the present-day catheterization technique of arteriography. This technique is the method of choice because of the following advantages over the percutaneous needle puncture method:[3] Multiple vessels including the aortic arch can be studied with only one arterial puncture; selective examinations are possible; the femoral or axillary artery puncture site for catheterization is remote from the important brachiocephalic arteries. If local complications occur at the puncture site, the major extracranial vessels are not affected; the catheter approach via the femoral artery is better tolerated by patients; multiple projections are facilitated by greater mobility and flexibility of the patient's head and neck; and the catheter technique has a much lower complication rate. The catheter technique, however, requires elaborate and expensive radiographic equipment, catheters, and guide wires, as well as skilled angiographers.

Percutaneous needle puncture of the carotid artery is rarely done. Indications usually include unsuccessful catheterization in the presence of tortuous brachiocephalic vessels and stenotic-occlusive vascular disease affecting the femoral and axillary arteries.

Radiographic Projections

For aortic arch studies, the right posterior oblique (35–45 degrees) is the single most informative projection. An anteroposterior and left posterior oblique view may also be necessary.

For the head and neck vessels, conventional anteroposterior and lateral views should include the cervical carotid and vertebral arteries as well as the intracranial circulation. A fluoroscopically positioned frontal oblique view of the common carotid bifurcation in patients with transient ischemic attacks or stroke is often necessary for a complete examination.

A prolonged angiographic series with delayed films is very important in differentiating between complete occlusion and near-complete occlusion of the internal carotid artery at its origin. A long segment of threadlike narrowing of the arterial lumen may otherwise be missed.[5]

Digital Subtraction Angiography (DSA)

Recent technologic advances in television, digital electronics, and image intensifier design with improved electronic recording of images has led to renewed interest in the technique of intravenous arteriography. Since the contrast medium is injected intravenously, the major risks of arterial injection are eliminated.[6] Some hospital centers are currently using intravenous DSA to evaluate aortic arch anomalies and the patency of vascular bypass grafts. In some centers it has replaced angiography in the evaluation of carotid bruits and nonspecific neurologic symptoms possibly caused by central nervous system ischemia or embolization, as well as the presurgical evaluation of extracranial brachiocephalic vessels in cardiac and coronary artery surgery patients with neck bruits.[6,7]

Complications

A decrease in the rate of complications of brachiocephalic arteriography has resulted from the change in technique from percutaneous needle puncture to catheterization, refinement of catheters and guidewires, improved contrast media, and an increase in the number of experienced angiographers. For all complications of angiography the rate has varied from 26.3 percent[8] to 0.9 percent.[9] These complications are local (at the puncture site), systemic (systems other than the CNS), and neurologic; they may be transient or permanent. The local and systemic complications are discussed in Chapter 5.

The rate of permanent neurologic complications has varied from 1.3 percent to none.[10,11] From a combination of seven separate series by various investigators, a mean rate of 0.59 percent permanent neurologic complications was reported.[12] The factors important for fewer complications are that the catheter be as small and as soft as possible (size 5F is preferable over larger sizes);[3,4] meglumine-bound iodinated contrast be used meglumine-bound medium causes fewer complications than sodium-bound iodine compounds;[13,14] the duration of the procedure be short (the shorter the duration, the lower the number of complications; procedures lasting over 80 minutes have a higher complication rate;[13] the patient be adequately hydrated (adequate hydration of the patient lowers the incidence of complications, especially systemic ones, such as renal failure and cardiac arrest);[3,4] and that the angiographers be experienced.[3,4,9]

RADIOGRAPHIC ANATOMY, VARIANTS, AND CONGENITAL ANOMALIES

The Aortic Arch

The brachiocephalic branches from a normal left aortic arch are the innominate, the left common carotid, and the left subclavian arteries. Occasionally the right subclavian artery originates as the last branch of the aortic arch. The aortic arch may arise from the right, in which case the vessels are a mirror image of the left arch, or may be duplicated, or may rarely extend into the neck as a cervical arch.[15,16]

The Innominate Artery

The innominate artery is the first branch of the aortic arch. It has a short trunk that terminates into the right common carotid and the right subclavian branches. The innominate artery is absent when the right subclavian artery or the right common carotid artery originates from the aortic arch.

The Subclavian Artery

The first segment of the subclavian artery from its origin to the scalenus anticus muscle will be considered in this chapter. Normally, the left subclavian artery is the last branch of the aortic arch, and the right subclavian artery is a branch of the innominate artery. The right subclavian artery may arise directly from the aortic arch as the first branch or the last branch distal to the origin of the left subclavian artery.[15,17] The left subclavian artery arising from the innominate artery or as a fourth vessel distal to the origin of the right subclavian may be seen with a right aortic arch.[15,18]

The first branch of the subclavian artery is the vertebral artery. The thyrocervical trunk and internal mammary artery also arise from the first part of the subclavian artery.

The Common Carotid Artery

While the right common carotid artery is a terminal branch of the innominate artery, the left common carotid artery arises directly from the aortic arch as its second branch. The common carotid artery terminates into the internal and external carotid branches at the carotid bifurcation, which is usually located about C-3 or C-4, but may be located as high as C-1 and as low as T-2.[15]

The right common carotid artery may originate directly from the aortic arch. Rarely, there is unilateral or bilateral absence of the common carotid artery with independent origins of the internal and external carotid arteries from the aortic arch. The anomaly is often associated with other major vascular anomalies.[19,20]

The Cervical Internal Carotid Artery

The paired cervical internal carotid arteries extend from the common carotid bifurcations to the skull base. At its origin, the internal carotid artery is usually lateral and posterior to the external carotid artery. The cervical internal carotid artery is usually straight, but it may have tortuosity in the form of coils, loops, and kinks. The loops and coils seen in children as well as adults are developmental, whereas the kinks, seen after third decade of life, have an unknown cause. The loops, coils and kinks of the carotid arteries usually do not have clinical significance.[21] Normally, the cervical internal carotid artery does not have branches, but the ascending pharyngeal, occipital, persistent hypoglossal or persistent proatlantal intersegmental arteries may arise as anomalous branches.[16]

Congenital absence of the internal carotid artery is rare and is associated with absence of the carotid canal within the petrous temporal bone.[22] Unilateral absence of the internal carotid artery is three times more frequent on the left than on the right. Congenital absence of the internal carotid artery is associated with an unusually high incidence of intracranial aneurysms.[22,23]

The internal carotid artery may be hypoplastic on one or both sides as a congenital anomaly occasionally associated with neurofibromatosis or anencephaly. Hypoplasia of the internal carotid artery associated with a small bony canal must be differentiated from diffuse narrowing of the artery in arteritis, spontaneous dissection, fibromuscular dysplasia, or marked proximal segmental stenosis with narrowed arterial lumen.[24]

The External Carotid Artery

Only the most proximal cervical segment of the external carotid artery will be considered in this chapter. The external carotid artery is the smaller of the terminal branches of the common carotid artery and supplies the face, scalp, cerebral dura mater, and superior part of the thyroid gland. The branches of the external carotid artery are the superior thyroid, the ascending pharyngeal, the lingual, the facial, the occipital, the posterior auricular, the superficial temporal, and the maxillary arteries.[25] The external carotid artery may arise directly from the aortic arch when the common carotid artery is absent.[19,20]

The Vertebral Artery

The vertebral artery is the first branch of the subclavian artery. After a variable distance from its origin, the vertebral artery ascends vertically through the transverse foramina from C-6 to C-2. It then courses backward and horizontally over the posterior arch of C-1. Finally it turns medially and superiorly to enter the skull through the foramen magnum, where it pierces the dura. The left vertebral artery may be larger than (42 percent), smaller than (32 percent), or approximately the same size as (26 percent) the right vertebral artery.[26]

The cervical vertebral artery gives rise to segmental muscular and radiculomedullary branches. There are anastomoses between the muscular branches of the vertebral artery and the occipital branch of the external carotid artery and between the segmental branches of the vertebral artery and the ascending pharyngeal artery, which is a branch of the external carotid artery.[27]

The left vertebral artery may arise from the aortic arch in 2 to 6 percent of cases. Either vertebral artery may originate as a branch of the innominate, the common carotid, or the external carotid artery. Bifid or duplicate origin of the left vertebral artery from the aortic arch and the subclavian artery is extremely rare.[28,29]

ABNORMALITIES OF THE BRACHIOCEPHALIC ARTERIES

Atherosclerosis

Atherosclerosis causes elongation, dilatation, and plaque formation, leading to stenosis, occlusion, and ulceration of the affected vessels. Subintimal hematoma in a plaque may cause abrupt narrowing of the arterial lumen.

THE CERVICAL CAROTID ARTERY

The most common sites of atherosclerotic changes involving the extracranial brachiocephalic vessels are the proximal internal carotid artery and the common carotid bifurcation. The proximal vertebral artery is the next most common site. In the majority of patients, multiple vessels and sites, including the intracranial vessels, are often involved.[30,31]

Stenosis of the internal carotid artery at its origin is considered marked or critical if the cross-sectional area of the residual lumen is less than 2 mm^2 or decreased by

70 percent.[32,33] Intraluminal thrombus distal to severe atherosclerotic stenosis at the origin of the internal carotid artery may be seen (Fig. 17-1). Such a thrombus may enlarge to occlude the vessel or embolize distally.[34] Severe stenosis with near total occlusion at the internal carotid artery origin may be mistaken for complete occlusion unless a long threadlike narrowed segment of the internal carotid artery is diligently sought for and confirmed by a long filming sequence, subtraction radiographs, and, if necessary, longer injection time.[12] Such apparent narrowing is due to incomplete filling of the vessel distal to near total occlusion (Fig. 17-2): it may mimic diffuse narrowing of the cervical internal carotid artery, neurofibromatosis, spontaneous dissection, arteritis, and recanalization of the artery following thrombosis. In spontaneous dissection, the stenosis of the internal carotid artery usually extends from the proximal internal carotid artery to the petrous canal.[35]

Ulceration of the atherosclerotic plaque may cause distal embolization, either by release of intraluminal cholesterol, platelet plugs, or fibrin clots. Platelets adhere, degranulate, and aggregate when they are exposed to subendothelial collagen and elastin in an ulcerated plaque (Fig. 17-3). These platelet aggregates may cause thrombosis in situ or distal embolization.[36] In a recent study, only 60 percent of ulcers in plaques seen at surgery were diagnosed at angiography.[37]

Spontaneous subintimal hemorrhage in an atherosclerotic plaque may cause symptoms because of sudden narrowing of the arterial lumen or distal embolization secondary to the rupture of the intima or endothelium. It is postulated that the hemorrhage is caused by spontaneous rupture of small dilated vessels within the plaque.[38] The typical radiographic appearance of such hemorrhage in an atheroma is a sharply marginated, rounded, eccentric filling defect. These lesions often simulate a smooth or ulcerated plaque.[38]

THE CERVICAL VERTEBRAL ARTERY

The proximal segment of the vertebral artery is the second most common site of stenotic or occlusive atherosclerotic lesions in the neck.[31]

THE SUBCLAVIAN ARTERY

Stenosis or occlusion of the subclavian or innominate artery proximal to the origin of the vertebral artery may produce a subclavian steal syndrome (Fig. 17-4). Atherosclerosis is the most common cause of subclavian steal. Less common causes are trauma, embolization, congenital anomalies, and therapeutic surgical procedures that cause stenosis or occlusion of the subclavian or innominate artery. Angiography documents occlusion or stenosis of the subclavian or innominate artery and delayed retrograde filling of the ipsilateral vertebral and subclavian arteries distal to the occlusion via the contralateral vertebral artery and the basilar artery, thus causing a steal of blood from the posterior fossa.[39] Sometimes angiographically demonstrated subclavian steal may be asymptomatic.[32,36]

Cervical Spondylosis

In severe spondylosis, a characteristic washboard appearance of the vertebral artery is created by multiple lateral convexities of the artery at the level of the intervertebral disc spaces, where bony osteophytes displace the artery laterally. Such lateral displacement is most common at the C4-5 and C5-6 intervertebral spaces.

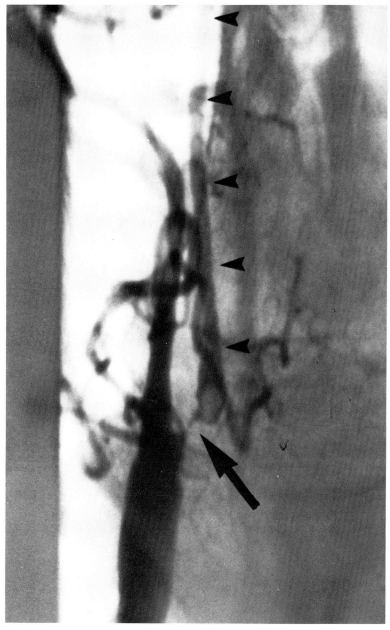

Figure 17-1. Anteroposterior-view carotid arteriogram demonstrates intraluminal clot just distal to marked internal carotid stenosis (arrow). The cervical internal carotid distal to the clot shows normal lumen (arrowheads).

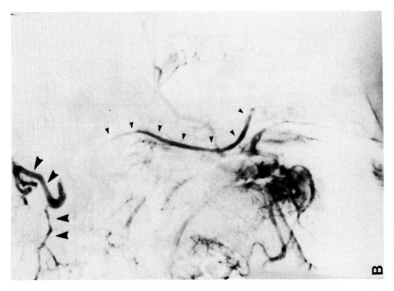

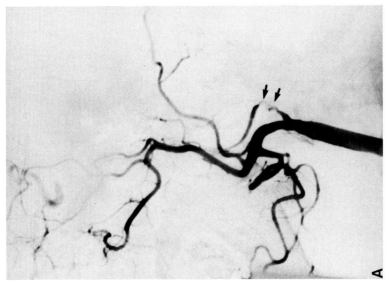

Figure 17-2. Common carotid arteriogram, early arterial phase (A) demonstrates near-total occlusion (arrows) of the internal carotid artery. Late arterial phase (B) shows delayed and incomplete filling (small arrowheads) of the internal carotid distal to the stenosis. The carotid siphon fills from the external carotid collaterals via the ophthalmic artery (large arrowheads).

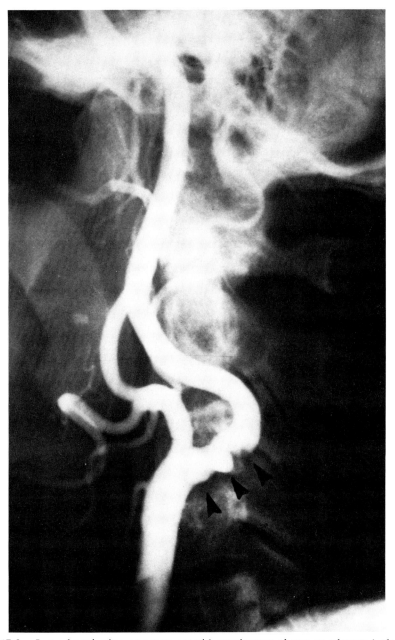

Figure 17-3. Lateral-projection common carotid arteriogram shows an ulcerated plaque at the internal carotid origin (arrowheads).

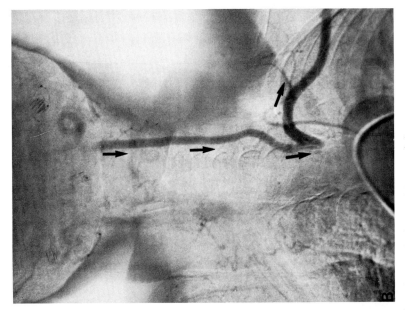

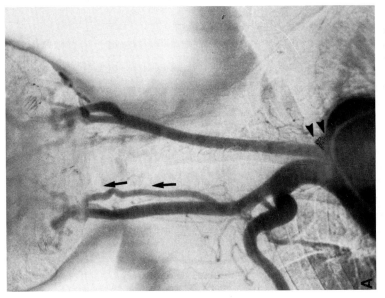

Figure 17-4. Arch aortogram demonstrating subclavian steal syndrome. Early arterial phase (A) shows complete occlusion of the left subclavian artery just beyond the origin (arrowheads). The right vertebral artery fills in normal antegrade fashion (arrows). Late arterial phase (B) shows retrograde filling of the left vertebral artery and the left subclavian artery (arrows).

Slight stenosis is frequent and occlusion rare at the point of lateral displacement. Since symptoms of vertebral ischemia may occur during rotation of the neck, angiography is performed in symptom-producing positions of the neck.[36,40,41]

Fibromuscular Dysplasia

Fibromuscular dysplasia is a disease of unknown etiology that affects the small- and medium-sized arteries. Cervical fibromuscular dysplasia typically involves the internal carotid artery or the vertebral artery at C1–C2 level; the lesions are usually bilateral. A high incidence of intracranial aneurysm has been noted with fibromuscular dysplasia. The most common angiographic finding is a typical "string of beads" appearance (80–85 percent) (Fig. 17-5). This appearance must be differentiated from stationary arterial waves, where the constrictions are more regularly spaced and occur without the intervening segmental dilatation seen in fibromuscular dysplasia.[42,43,44] The stationary waves usually occur proximal to a site of partial or complete arterial obstruction and are probably caused by rapid injection of contrast media.[45]

A less frequently seen pattern is tubular stenosis (6–12 percent), which has to be differentiated from congenital arterial hypoplasia, arteritis, vascular spasm, spontaneous arterial dissection, and near-complete vascular occlusion.[44]

A diverticulum-like outpouching from one wall of the artery has been classified as atypical fibromuscular dysplasia (4–6 percent). Such atypical appearance may mimic atherosclerotic or posttraumatic aneurysm.[43,44] Rarely, fibromuscular dysplasia also involves intracranial vessels. The disease may be progressive, and patients with craniocervical fibromuscular dysplasia may have significant cerebrovascular symptoms.[44,46]

Arteritis

Stenotic and occlusive lesions may be produced by various types of arteritis. Takayasu's arteritis (pulseless disease, aortic arch syndrome, aortitis syndrome) is a disease of unknown etiology that primarily involves the aorta and its branches in young women. Angiograms of the brachiocephalic vessels show fusiform stenosis of variable length that begins at the origin of one or more vessels.[47,48]

Giant cell arteritis (cranial arteritis, temporal arteritis, or granulomatous arteritis) typically involves external carotid and ophthalmic arteries. Postmortem studies have shown severe involvement of the cervical vertebral arteries in a high proportion of cases. In these postmortem studies, the cervical internal carotid arteries were less frequently involved by giant cell arteritis, and the pathological changes were mild. Lesions may also be seen at the carotid siphon and the distal vertebral arteries where these vessels penetrate the dura mater.[49]

Vascular Trauma

Arteriography is the method of choice for the detection of traumatic lesions of the brachiocephalic arteries. Penetrating or blunt trauma may result in vascular damage to one or more vessels. Penetrating injuries may result from stabs, missiles, inadvertent laceration at surgery, or from direct needle puncture arteriography.[50] Blunt vascular trauma may be direct or indirect. Direct blunt injuries are caused by trauma to the neck or chest or intraoral foreign bodies. Indirect blunt injuries are usually associated

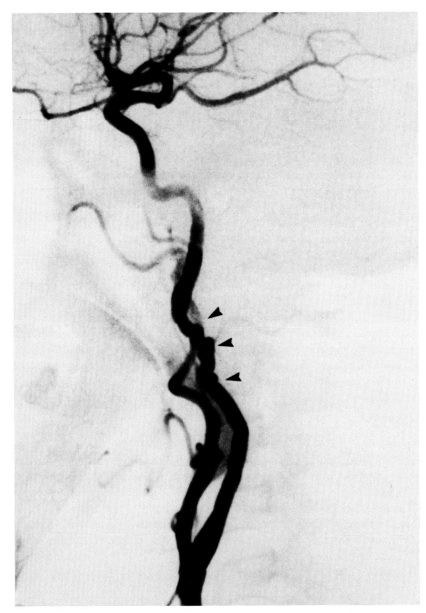

Figure 17-5. Common carotid arteriogram shows typical "string of beads" appearance (arrowheads) of fibromuscular dysplasia of the internal carotid artery at C-1 and C-2 level.

with head trauma. Penetrating or blunt vascular trauma may cause symptoms as a result of intimal tear, thrombosis, occlusion, stenosis, pseudoaneurysm (Fig. 17-6), or arteriovenous fistula.[50]

Unlike the vertebral artery, which courses through the bony transverse canal, the cervical carotid artery is relatively unprotected and is the vessel most often involved in injury. Most of the blunt traumatic lesions are caused by vehicular accidents and typically involve the carotid artery 1 to 3 cm above the common carotid bifurcation.[51,52]

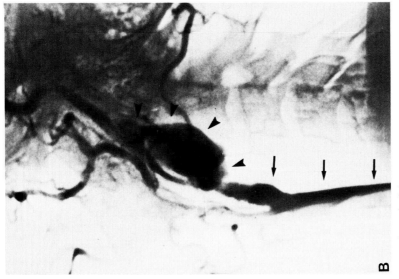

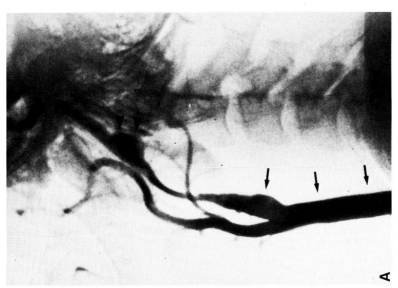

Figure 17-6. Pseudoaneurysm of the internal carotid artery and cervical hematoma from a stab wound. Early arterial phase (A) shows anterior displacement of the common and internal carotid arteries (arrows). Narrowing of the internal carotid and partial filling of the pseudoaneurysm (arrowheads) are seen. Later radiograph in midarterial phase (B) demonstrates completely filled pseudoaneurysm (arrowheads). [Courtesy of Lewis Segal, MD, Chicago, Ill.]

Such lesions should be clinically suspected and angiographically confirmed in conscious patients with an onset of focal neurologic deficit several hours after injury, a Horner's syndrome, or cervical hematoma with a normal cranial computed tomographic scan.[52,53]

The third segment of the vertebral artery extending from C-1 to its entry into the skull is particularly vulnerable to injuries resulting from rotation, hyperextension, and tilting of the head. This segment of the vertebral artery is relatively fixed and located around the mobile atlantoaxial joint. Traumatic lesions of the vertebral artery have been caused by chiropractic or neck manipulation, minor falls, automobile accidents, yoga or gymnastic exercises, ceiling painting, archery practice, and spontaneous head turning while driving an automobile.[41,54,55]

Aneurysms

Aneurysms of the cervical carotid artery are uncommon. The common causes of such aneurysms are arteriosclerosis, trauma, congenital or developmental defects, and infection.[56]

Aneurysms of the extracranial vertebral artery are rare. The second segment of the vertebral artery from C-6 to C-1 is the most common site (70 percent). In most instances, these aneurysms are secondary to trauma. Enlargement of the neural foramina has been reported with these aneurysms.[28]

Arteriovenous Communications

Arteriovenous communications of the neck vessels will usually involve the vertebral artery (Fig. 17-7). A traumatic arteriovenous fistula of the vertebral artery is more often encountered than is a congenital arteriovenous malformation. Such arteriovenous communications are often supplied by both vertebral arteries and may have contributions from the external carotid artery branches and the internal carotid artery via the circle of Willis.[28,57]

Neoplasms

The cervical internal carotid artery may be displaced by paragangliomas (Fig. 17-8), neurofibromas, enlarged lymph nodes, thyroid masses, brachial cleft cysts, and cystic hygromas. Infiltrating neoplasms may displace, compress, and occlude the cervical carotid artery.[24,58]

The cervical segment of the vertebral artery is unlikely to be displaced because of its location within the transverse foramina. Meningeal, radicular, and muscular branches of the vertebral artery may contribute to the vascular supply of meningiomas, neurofibromas, paragangliomas, and hemangioblastomas of the spinal cord.[59]

ACKNOWLEDGMENTS

The author is grateful for the invaluable editorial comments of Dr. Bertram Levin. He is also thankful to Margaret J. Lappin for typing the manuscript.

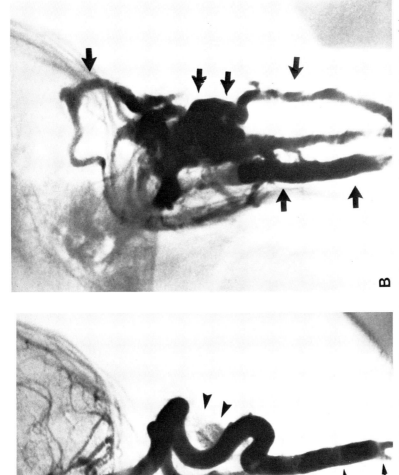

Figure 17-7. Laterial-view vertebral arteriograms demonstrate arteriovenous communication. Early arterial phase (A) shows enlarged vertebral arteries (arrows) and early filling of an enlarged cervical vein (arrowheads). Mid-arterial phase (B) demonstrates numerous dilated cervical veins (arrows).

319

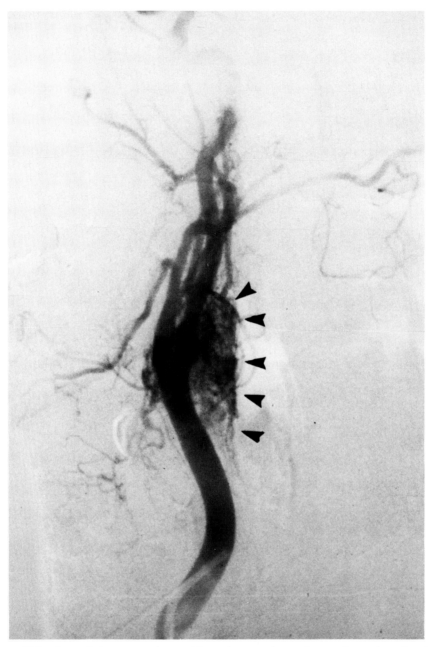

Figure 17-8. Lateral-view common carotid arteriogram shows abnormal vessels and stain of a carotid paraganglioma (arrowheads). [Courtesy of Tulsi Sawlani, MD, Valparaiso, Ind.]

REFERENCES

1. Barnes RW, Liebman PR, Marszalek PB, et al: The natural history of asymptomatic carotid disease in patients undergoing cardiovascular surgery. Surgery 90:1075–1083, 1981

2. Greenberger P, Patterson R, Kelly J, et al: Administration of radiographic contrast media in high risk patients. Invest Radiol 15:540–543, 980

3. Newton TH, Kerber CW: Techniques of cerebral angiography, in Newton TH, Potts DG (eds): Radiology of Skull and Brain; vol 2. St. Louis, C.V. Mosby, 1974, pp 920–938

4. Kerber CW, Cromwell LD, Drayer BP, et al: Cerebral ischemia. 1. Current angiographic techniques, complications, and safety. AJR 130:1097–1103, 1978

5. Gabrielsen TO, Seeger JF, Knake JE, et al: The nearly occluded internal carotid artery: A diagnostic trap. Radiology 138:611–618, 1981

6. Mistretta CA, Crummy AB, Strother CM: Digital angiography: A perspective. Radiology 139:273–276, 1981

7. Chilcote WA, Modic MT, Pavlicek WA, et al: Digital subtraction angiography of the carotid arteries: A comparative study in 100 patients. Radiology 139:287–295, 1981

8. Olivecrona H: Complications of cerebral angiography. Neuroradiology 14:175–181, 1977

9. Mani RL, Eisenberg RL, McDonald EJ, et al: Complications of catheter cerebral arteriography: Analysis of 5000 procedures. 1. Criteria and incidence. AJR 131:861–865, 1978

10. Wishart DL: Complications in vertebral angiography as compared to nonvertebral cerebral angiography in 447 studies. AJR 113:527–537, 1971

11. Eisenberg RL, Bank WO, Hedgecock MW: Neurologic complications of angiography for cerebrovascular disease. Neurology 30:895–897, 1980

12. Huckman MS, Shenk GI, Neems RL, et al: Transfemoral cerebral arteriography versus direct percutaneous carotid and brachial arteriography: A comparison of complication rates. Radiology 132:93–97, 1979

13. Mani RL, Eisenberg RL: Complications of catheter cerebral arteriography: Analysis of 5,000 procedures. III. Assessment of arteries injected, contrast medium used, duration of procedure and age of patient. AJR 131:871–874, 1978

14. Fischer HW: Contrast media, in Newton TH, Potts DG (eds): Radiology of the Skull and Brain, vol. 1. St. Louis, C.V. Mosby, 1974, pp 893–907

15. Haughton VM, Rosenbaum AE: The normal and anomalous aortic arch and brachiocephalic arteries, in Newton TH, Potts DG (eds): Radiology of the Skull and Brain, vol 2. St. Louis, C.V. Mosby, 1974, pp 1145–1163

16. Osborn AG: The aortic arch and its branches, in Introduction to Cerebral Angiography. Hagerstown, Harper & Row, 1980, pp 33–48

17. Boechat MI, Gilsanz V, Fellows KE: Subclavian artery as the first branch of the aortic arch: A normal variant in two patients. AJR 131:721–722, 1978

18. Nath PH, Castaneda-Zuniga W, Zollikofer CL, et al: An unusual aberrant left subclavian artery. Radiology 143:17–18, 1980

19. Bryan RN, Drewyer RG, Gee W: Separate origins of the left internal and external carotid arteries from the aorta. AJR 130:362–365, 1978

20. Roberts LK, Gerald B: Absence of both common carotid arteries. AJR 130:981–982, 1978

21. Asamoah DK, Foy PM: Some radiological abnormalities of the cervical carotid artery and their clinical significance. Clin Radiol 30:593–599, 1979

22. Teal JS, Naheedy MH, Hasso AN: Total agenesis of the internal carotid artery. AJNR 1:435–442, 1980

23. Servo A: Agenesis of the left internal carotid artery associated with an aneurysm on the right carotid syphon. J Neurosurg 46:677–680, 1977

24. Osborn AG: The internal carotid artery: Cervical and petrous portions, in Introduction to Cerebral Angiography. Hagerstown, Harper & Row, 1980, pp 87–108

25. Salamon G, Faure J, Raybaud C, et al: The external carotid artery, in Newton TH, Potts DG (eds): Radiology of the Skull and Brain, vol 2. St. Louis, C.V. Mosby, 1974, pp 1246–1274

26. Taveras JM, Wood EH: Vertebral Angiography. In Robbins LL (ed): Golden's Diagnostic Radiology, Section 1, Vol 2. Baltimore, Williams & Wilkins, 1976, pp 778–848

27. Lasjaunias P, Manelfe C: Arterial supply for the upper cervical nerves and the cervicocarotid anastomotic channels. Neuroradiology 18:125–131, 1979

28. Newton TH, Mani RL: The vertebral artery, in Newton TH, Potts DG (eds): Radiology of the Skull and Brain, vol. 2. St. Louis, C.V. Mosby, 1974, pp 1659–1709

29. Suzuki S, Kuwabara Y, Hatano R, et al: Duplicate origin of left vertebral artery. Neuroradiology 15:27–29, 1978

30. Hass WK, Fields WS, North RR, et al: Joint study of extracranial arterial occlusions. II: Arteriography, techniques, sites, and complications. JAMA 203:961–968, 1968

31. Kilgore BB, Fields WS: Arterial occlusive disease in adults, in Newton TH, Potts DG (eds): Radiology of the Skull and Brain, vol 2. St. Louis, C.V. Mosby, 1974, pp 2310–2343

32. Heilbrun MP: Transient cerebral ischemia: Surgical considerations. Progr Cardiovasc Dis 22:378–388, 1980

33. Brice JG, Dowsett DJ, Lowe RD: Hemodynamic effects of carotid artery stenosis. Br Med J 2:1363–1366, 1964

34. Roberson GH, Scott WR, Rosenbaum AE: Thrombi at the site of carotid stenosis. Radiology 109:353–356, 1973

35. O'Dwyer JA, Moscow N, Trevor R: Spontaneous dissection of the carotid artery. Radiology 137:379–385, 1980

36. Schmidley JW, Caronna JJ: Transient cerebral ischemia: Pathophysiology. Progr Cardiovasc Dis 22:325–342, 1980

37. Edwards JH, Kricheff II, Riles T, et al: Angiographically undetected ulceration of the carotid bifurcation as a cause of embolic stroke. Radiology 132:369–373, 1979

38. Edwards JH, Kricheff II, Gorstein F, et al: Atherosclerotic subintimal hematoma of the carotid artery. Radiology 133:123–129, 1979

39. Bohmfalk GL, Story JL, Brown WE, et al: Subclavian steal syndrome. J Neurosurg 51:618–640, 1979

40. Sheehan S, Bauer RB, Meyer JS: Vertebral artery compression in cervical spondylosis. Neurology 10:968–986, 1960

41. Caplan LR: Patterns of Posterior Circulation infarction and correlation with vascular pathology. In Baur R, Berger R (eds): Vertebrobasilar Arterial Occlusive Disease. Medical and Surgical Management. Proceedings of the First International Conference. Raven Press, New York, 1983 (in press)

42. Palubinskas AJ, Perloff D, Newton TH: Fibromuscular hyperplasia: An arterial dysplasia of increasing clinical importance. AJR 98:907–913, 1966

43. Houser OW, Baker HL: Fibromuscular dysplasia and other uncommon diseases of the cervical carotid artery: Angiographic aspects. AJR 104:201–212, 1968

44. Osborn AG, Anderson RD: Angiographic spectrum of cervical and intracranial fibromuscular dysplasia. Stroke 8:617–626, 1977

45. New PF: Arterial stationary waves. AJR 97:488–499, 1966

46. Corrin LS, Sandok BA, Houser OW: Cerebral ischemic events in patients with carotid artery fibromuscular dysplasia. Arch Neurol 38:616–618, 1981

47. Ferris EJ: Arteritis, in Newton TH, Potts DG (eds): Radiology of Skull and Brain, vol. 2. St. Louis, C.V. Mosby, 1974, pp 2566–2597

48. Lande A, Rossi P: The value of total aortography in the diagnosis of Takayasu's arteritis. Radiology 114:287–297, 1975

49. Wilkinson LM, Russel RW: Arteries of the head and neck in giant cell arteritis: A pathological study to show the pattern of arterial involvement. Arch Neurol 27:378–391, 1972

50. Stringer WL, Kelly DL: Traumatic dissection of the extracranial internal carotid artery. Neurosurgery 6:123–130, 1980

51. Sullivan HG, Vines FS, Becker DP: Sequelae of indirect internal carotid injury. Radiology 109:91–98, 1973

52. Krajewski LP, Hertner NR: Blunt carotid artery trauma: Report of two cases and review of the literature. Ann Surg 191:341–346, 1980

53. French BN, Cobb CA, Dublin AB: Cranial computed tomography in the diagnosis of symptomatic indirect trauma to the carotid artery. Surg Neurol 15:256–267, 1981

54. Robertson JT: Editorial: Neck manipulation as a cause of stroke. Stroke 12:1, 1981

55. Sherman DG, Hart RG, Easton JD: Abrupt change in head position and cerebral infarction. Stroke 12:2–6, 1981

56. Margolis MT, Stein RL, Newton TH: Extracranial aneurysms of the internal carotid artery. Neuroradiology 4:78–89, 1972

57. Lawson TL, Newton TH: Congenital cervical arteriovenous malformations. Radiology 97:565–570, 1970

58. Dilenge D, Maurice H: The internal carotid artery, in Newton TH, Potts DG (eds): Radiology of Skull and Brain, vol. 2. St. Louis, C.V. Mosby, 1974, pp 1201–1245

59. Osborn AG: Arteries and veins of the posterior fossa, in Introduction to Cerebral Angiography. Hagerstown, Harper & Row, 1980, pp 379–427

Janice R.L. Smith
Gerald D. Pond

18

Digital Subtraction Angiography of the Carotid Arteries

Chapter 7 covered the technical aspects of digital subtraction angiography. This chapter will deal with its application to the evaluation of the carotid arteries.

TECHNIQUE

All of our early work[1-4] was done with a 9-inch intensifier. The recent addition of a 14.5-inch intensifier on a second C-arm has expanded the field of view of our system while still offering higher resolution modes of 10-inch and 6-inch fields. Ultimately it is hoped that both these intensifiers will be used for biplane imaging.

The standard carotid examination includes four views (Fig. 18-1): frontal and two oblique views of the cervical vessels and a frontal view of the intracranial vasculature. The full 14.5-inch field is used on the initial run. The patient's torso is positioned obliquely to the right to open up the aortic arch, but the head is not turned in order to obtain a frontal view of the cervical carotids. With this one projection, the innominate, proximal subclavian, common carotid, external carotid, cervical internal carotid, and cervical vertebral arteries can all be screened simultaneously.

This first projection demonstrates the relative position of each internal carotid to its corresponding external carotid artery and of the cervical carotid vessels to the ipsilateral vertebral artery. This information helps in determining the ideal degree of obliquity to open each common carotid artery bifurcation. Note that in Figure 18-1A, while the left internal carotid artery takes the usual position lateral to the left external carotid artery, the proximal right internal carotid lies slightly medial to the right external carotid artery. From this first view it could be predicted that the right posterior oblique projection would not only open up the left common carotid artery bifurcation but also the right. This is confirmed in Figure 18-1B. With experience,

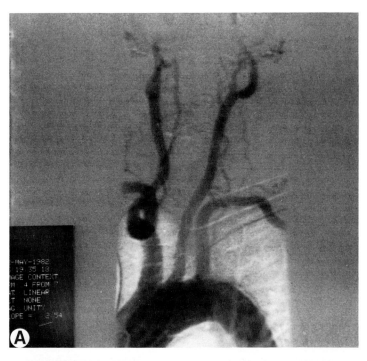

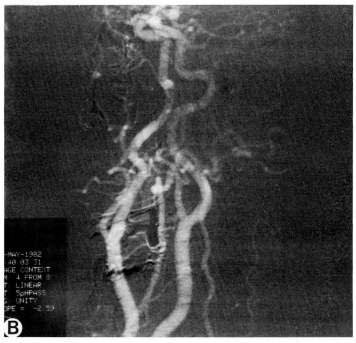

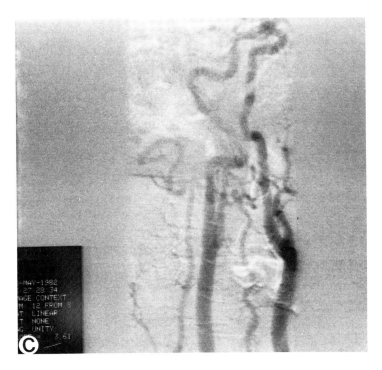

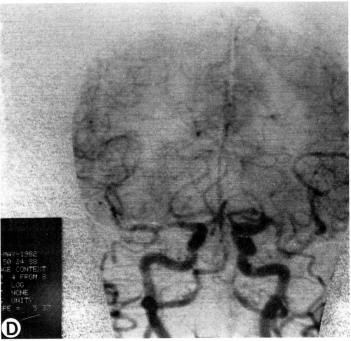

Figure 18-1. Standard carotid artery examination. (A) Initial arch and neck projection. (B, C) Right and left oblique views of carotid bifurcations including the entire internal carotid arteries. (D) Frontal intracranial study.

skill and, occasionally, luck, the internal and external carotid arteries usually can be adequately separated without obscuring the area of interest with a superimposed vertebral artery. The oblique views are performed with the 10-inch mode of the 14.5-inch intensifier, which provides a large enough field of view to include not only the common carotid artery bifurcation but also the juxtasellar portions of the internal carotid arteries. Before this capability was available there was little chance of detecting stenoses in the carotid system. The fourth view of this standard examination is a frontal intracranial view, which provides a survey of the intracranial circulation.

Some attention must be given to a few impediments often encountered. Intravenous digital subtraction angiography in the head and neck region presents some additional difficulties in collimation and technique selection compared with more uniform regions such as the abdomen. There is a wide range of x-ray absorption to be dealt with between the soft tissues of the neck and the dense base of skull and within the cylindrical neck with tapering tissue volume laterally and dense vertebral bodies more centrally. The soft tissue densities can be made more uniform by the addition of water or flour bags laterally. This can also be helpful over the apices of the lung. We are now experimenting with plexiglass wedge filters of varying shapes, which can be positioned on the collimator. Use of the square root function for data acquisition also allows wider ranges of density to be satisfactorily examined. For the intracranial projection, a lead template is affixed to the intensifier and manipulated to compliment the curvature of the cranial vault.

Another difficulty is the simultaneous flooding of the entire arterial system. The problem of overlapping vessels can necessitate additional views, but there is not much leeway on this point, since there is a limit to the volume of contrast that can be safely administered.

Decreased cardiac output results in a dilution and prolongation of the contrast bolus. Both result in less contrast for each image and, therefore, a degradation of image quality.

The most common and most severe problem is patient motion. This technique is critically dependent on patient immobility. Even slight motion of the head can significantly degrade the final image. Respiration during imaging of the neck and upper chest will also produce a poor subtraction image. Swallowing is a most disruptive sort of motion, especially on the oblique views of the neck, and, unfortunately, most contrast agents now available for intravenous use are known to induce the urge to swallow when delivered in bolus form. The variety of tricks conjured up to prevent swallowing attests to the significance of this problem. Our favorite is to tell the patient to hold the tip of the tongue pressed against the teeth (or gums). To reduce motion in general we use two Velcro straps, one across the forehead and one under the chin. For the intracranial run on patients who have shown some tendency to move, we use a head immobilizer developed here.[5] The patient makes a dental (or gingival) impression in a dental impression compound that has been molded around a bite bar. This bar is affixed to the stationary, boxlike head immobilizer (Fig. 18-2). If the patient bites steadily on the dental impression through the study, any motion, especially rotatory, should be eliminated. In some patients, a cough reflex is induced by the bolus injection. Head and neck imaging is impossible in those cases. The availability of intravenous contrast materials that do not produce discomfort, sensations of heat, or the urge to swallow or cough is eagerly awaited. At present, the best chance for success comes from communicating to the patient the importance of his or her immobility and absolute dependence on his or her cooperation.

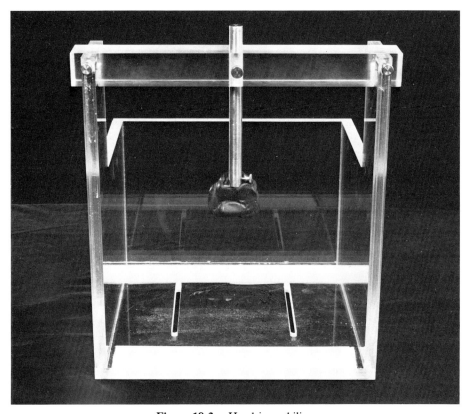

Figure 18-2.   Head immobilizer.

RESULTS

In the first 2 years of clinical use of our digital subtraction system, 303 patients were studied primarily to evaluate the cervical carotid arteries for atherosclerotic disease. These patients ranged in age from 33 to 87 years with a mean of 67.3 years and a median of 68 years. The most frequently encountered age was 71 years (15 patients). The ratio of males to females was 2 to 1.

Diagnostic studies were obtained in 94 percent of these cases. The most common reason for a suboptimal result was patient motion, as was previously discussed. Poor cardiac output and technical problems accounted for a smaller number of the failures.

Clearly there are numerous ways in which atherosclerotic disease of the carotid arteries can appear. Approximately one third of our patients had episodes consistent with transient ischemic attacks, and a smaller additional group had amaurosis fugax. The next largest group was made up of patients who had completed cerebrovascular accidents (CVAs). In general, these patients had recovered significantly from their CVAs, and an etiology was being sought in hopes of preventing future episodes. Roughly 15 percent of the cases were to be done because of a new or changing carotid artery bruit. Another group of patients, representing approximately 10 percent of these studies, fell within the broad category of cerebrovascular insufficiency. Some patients with known atherosclerotic disease (peripheral or coronary artery) were studied before their planned vascular surgery as a screen for significant lesions. If high-grade stenotic lesions of the cervical carotid arteries were found, carotid endarterec-tomies might then be indicated as the first operative procedure.

A comparative study of intraarterial and intravenous carotid angiography was performed by Chilcote et al.,[6] which showed excellent correlation between the two studies when the digital studies were of good quality. The image in Figure 18-3 demonstrates the difficulties that can be encountered with even a slight degree of motion. The vertebral column is not quite so well subtracted as it was in Figure 18-1. There is definitely atherosclerotic plaque in the distal right common carotid artery extending into the proximal internal carotid artery. There is a strong suggestion of an outpouching of contrast consistent with an ulceration in the plaque. This finding is somewhat cast in doubt by the misregistration of the bony subtraction resulting in a lucent line crossing just proximal to the apparent ulcer. It is easy to see why the highest quality images must be obtained in order to yield accurate diagnoses.

The issue is much more clear cut in Figure 18-4. Magnified views of a frontal and oblique projection clearly demonstrate atherosclerotic plaques in the left distal common and proximal internal carotid artery. This is producing at least a moderate stenosis, and a definite ulcer crater is seen. Fortunately it is these larger and more easily identified ulcer craters that are generally managed with surgery. The shallower,

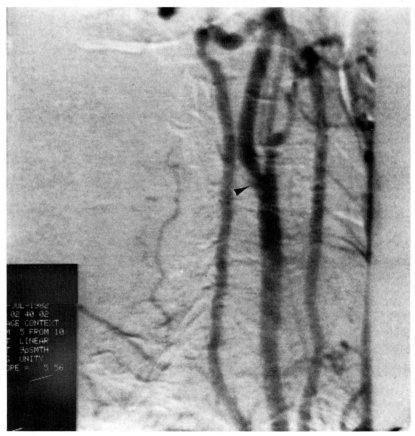

Figure 18-3. Atherosclerotic plaque of the right common carotid artery bifurcation with possible ulceration (arrowhead).

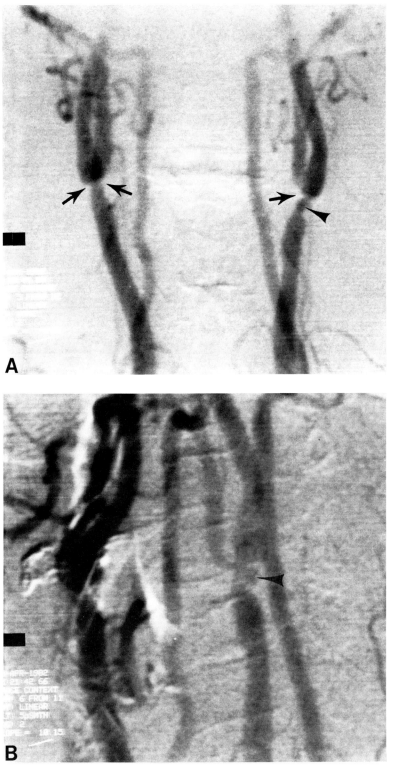

Figure 18-4. (A) Bilateral stenosis of the common carotid artery bifurcations (arrows). (B) An ulcer crater on the left (arrowhead).

more subtle ones can be missed by both intravenous and intraarterial angiography. These patients, however, are more likely to be placed on antiplatelet therapy on the basis of their symptoms even if minor irregularities are delineated angiographically.

Our level of confidence is generally very high in the diagnosis of significant stenosis or complete occlusion. In Figure 18-5, there is a very high grade stenosis of the proximal right internal carotid artery. Only a thin, somewhat irregular string of contrast is seen in the region of this large atherosclerotic plaque. There is a mild-to-moderate stenosis seen at the same level of the left internal carotid artery as well. Complete occlusion of the left internal carotid artery associated with an area of high-grade stenosis of the distal left common carotid artery is seen in Figure 18-6A. The surgical clips were introduced at the time of a carotid endarterectomy. The vertebro-basilar system is well demonstrated and the solitary right distal internal carotid artery nicely demonstrated with no superimposition of the left internal carotid artery.

The intracranial image in Figure 18-6B shows good filling of the left middle cerebral artery vessels via collateral flow. Serial intracranial images in cases of unilateral high-grade stenosis or occlusion of an internal carotid artery often reveal a delay in appearance and washout of contrast on the affected side. Sometimes the dominant source of the collateral supply from the opposite anterior cerebral artery, the ipsilateral

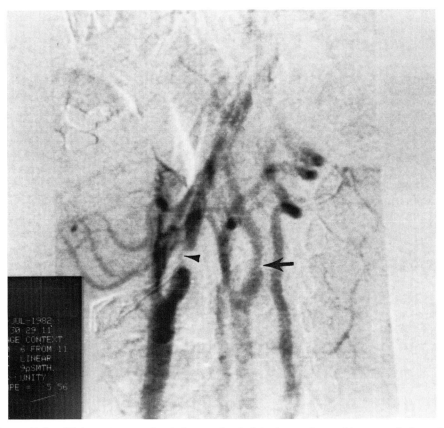

Figure 18-5. High-grade stenosis of the proximal right internal carotid artery. Only a thin strand of contrast material (arrowhead) is seen in this region. Minor atherosclerotic plaque can be seen in the proximal left internal carotid artery (arrow).

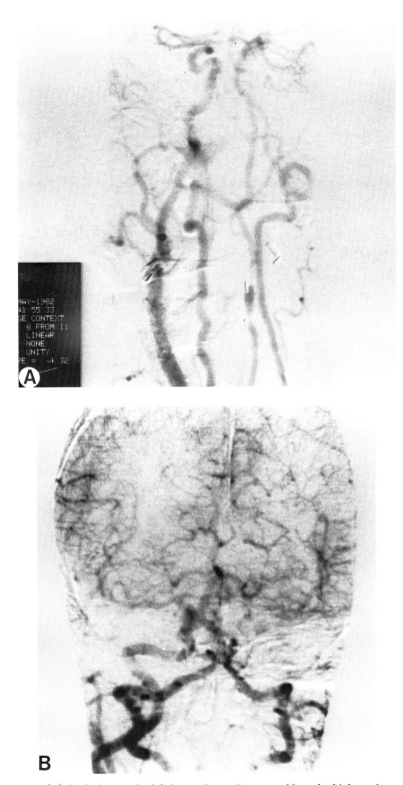

Figure 18-6. (A) Occlusion to the left internal carotid artery. Note the high-grade stenosis of the distal left common carotid artery. (B) Collateral flow supplies the left anterior and middle cerebral artery territories.

posterior communicating artery, or leptomeningeal flow is suggested. We are just beginning to analyze our data on this topic to see whether the intracranial studies may supply useful hemodynamic information. In several cases the intracranial series have delineated pertinent lesions such as stenoses or occlusions of the middle or posterior cerebral arteries. Of course, there are many applications for intracranial intravenous digital studies, but they go beyond the scope of this particular work.

THE CHOICE: INTRAARTERIAL OR INTRAVENOUS DIGITAL SUBTRACTION ANGIOGRAPHY?

The choice between an intraarterial or an intravenous approach is not always an easy or obvious decision to make because so many factors come into play. In general, in the case of an emergency such as crescendo transient ischemic attacks, we recommend the intraarterial approach. If the intravenous study was inconclusive for any reason, not only would time have been lost but the patient would have received a significant amount of contrast before the conventional angiogram. In nonemergent situations, however, the use of intravenous digital subtraction angiography is steadily expanding. As was discussed earlier, the radiologist is entirely dependent on the patients for their cooperation. If the patient is alert and cooperative, has satisfactory cardiac output, and can hold his or her breath for 20 seconds, the radiologist should be able to produce diagnostic images. Patients who do not meet these criteria are probably better suited for intraarterial study. There are always extenuating circumstances, however. We will often attempt a marginal case when there is a cogent reason to avoid the conventional study. For instance, a patient with known severe atherosclerotic peripheral vascular disease is clearly at an increased risk of cerebral infarction as a complication of intraarterial catheterization. In these and other cases, the intravenous approach may be tried first with the hope that we will succeed.

The real proof of digital subtraction angiography for carotid disease came when the surgeons started operating on the basis of the digital results alone, rather than simply using it as a screening technique to be followed later by conventional angiography. As a general rule, they are now very confident when shown an area of stenosis. They also feel comfortable with well-defined ulcerations such as in Figure 18-4. They are less likely to accept the ulcer shown in Figure 18-3 without additional proof. They seem most uncomfortable with the symptomatic patients in which no evidence of plaque is found. Whether a lesion was overlooked becomes the question. Recognizing the serious responsibility the vascular surgeon assumes in deciding whether or not to recommend surgery to a patient, we rarely hesitate to do a conventional study when the surgeon is not comfortable with the intravenous examination. It has been gratifying, however, to see that as all of us gain in experience with this new technique, fewer patients require both modalities.

REFERENCES

1. Carmody RF, Smith JRL, Seeger JF: Intravenous cerebral angiography: Early clinical experience. Ariz Med 38:349–350, 1981
2. Hillman BJ, Smith JRL, Pond GD, et al: Pho-
toelectronic radiology in Hanafee WN, Wilson GH (eds): Current Radiology, vol 4. New York, John Wiley & Sons, 1982
3. Pond GD, Smith JRL, Hillman BJ, et al: Cur-

rent clinical applications of digital video subtraction angiography. Appl Radiol 10:71–79,
1981

4. Seeger JF, Carmody RF, Smith JRL, et al: Digital intravenous cerebral angiography. Proc Soc
Photo-Opt Instr Eng 314:239–243, 1981

5. Seeger JF, Smith JRL, Carmody RF: Head im-

mobilizer for digital subtraction angiography.
AJNR 3:352–353, 982

6. Chilcote WA, Modic MT, Pavlicek MS, et al:
Digital subtraction angiography of the carotid
arteries: A comparative study in 100 patients.
Radiology 139:287–295, 1981

Index

SUTTER GENERAL HOSPITAL
NUCLEAR MEDICINE DEPARTMENT
2820 L STREET
SACRAMENTO, CA 95816

SUTTER GENERAL HOSPITAL
NUCLEAR MEDICINE DEPARTMENT
2820 L STREET
SACRAMENTO, CA 95816